Confessions of a

HEALER

Confessions *of a*

HEALER

THE TRUTH FROM AN

UNCONVENTIONAL

FAMILY DOCTOR

O.T. BONNETT, M.D.

MacMurray & Beck

Aspen, Colorado

Printed and bound in the United States of America.
Library of Congress Catalog Card Number: 94-077375

Library of Congress Cataloging-in-Publication Data

Bonnett, O. T., 1925-
    Confessions of a healer : the truth from an unconventional
family doctor / by O.T. Bonnett.
        p.   cm.
    ISBN 1-878448-61-7 : $18.95
    1. Alternative medicine. 2. Family medicine.
3. Psychophysiology. 4. Hypnotism--Therapeutic use. I. Title.
RS33.B66 1994
616'.001'9--dc20   94-26287
                                                            CIP

Book designed by Susan Wasinger, Boulder, Colorado

To my colleagues

who would have the courage

to be healers

CONTENTS

Wisdom cannot be communicated.

BUDDHA

PREFACE

This book was conceived over forty years ago. But only now have I felt I had the experience and maturity to write it. The ideas and concepts I have addressed are ones I firmly believe the public already understands—not necessarily in the framework in which I have presented them, but deep within its own level of awareness. Perhaps hearing those same beliefs expressed by a physician will strike a note of concurrence.

The book is the presentation of my, perhaps unconventional, views, based upon what I learned while conducting my practice. Threaded throughout the chapters is a recurring plea for patients to accept responsibility for their welfare. I am quite certain that when individuals give up their right to think for themselves and hand that right over to another individual or group, be it a doctor, government, church, or any other self-serving institution, they become less well off in the process.

My professional life was spent teaching wellness while trying to lead my patients toward a fuller understanding of self-realization. It is my desire that through this book I might reach others and share with them the benefit of my experience as a teacher, physician, and healer.

There are a number of different individuals I wish to thank. They have stood like beacons at pivotal points in my life, leading, pointing, and sometimes shoving me in the direction I was to take. They are, in no special order:

DR. HANS SELYE, whose work concerning the mechanisms by which chronic stress produces disease gave me untold hours of pleasure as I integrated his ideas into my thinking and previously held scientific beliefs.

DR. MICHAEL BALINT, for his understanding of the cooperative effort between the doctor and the patient in organizing an illness.

DAVE ELMAN, my hypnosis teacher, for expanding my understanding of the subconscious mind, its power over the physical body, and its relation to wellness and disease.

KARLFRIED GRAF VON DURKHEIM, who played a pivotal role early in my career, opening my mind to the concepts of Zen and the universal truths of all religions.

DR. PHIL KESSLER, my dear friend, who exposed me to the wonders of optometry, neurological development, and the concepts of space perception. He was a monument of integrity to be admired and emulated when my peers so often lacked that quality.

DRS. THERON RANDOLPH AND WILLIAM PHILPOTT are true pioneers in the field of ecologically induced diseases. The world owes them a vote of appreciation for their work and their persistence in the face of constant challenge and opposition.

DR. GEORGE GOODHEART, who introduced me to chiropractic and kinesiology and changed my bigoted attitude toward his approach to health care.

DR. DAN ALEXANDER, who taught me about TMJ syndrome and the importance of oral health to the well-being of the total person.

DR. JAMES DABNEY, who led me to the wonders of acupuncture and further opened my mind to the concept of man as an energy field.

JEFF MORRIS, my friend and psychic, who helped me recall many of my previous incarnations and introduced me to my spiritual guide.

DR. RALPH WARNER, who has done more for me than I can relate. Ralph and his guide, Hector, have given me much assistance, help, comfort, and knowledge through our many years of friendship.

GREG SATRE has been like a son and at the same time a teacher to me. A gifted psychic, he has contributed much to this book. It is through his urging that this book was finally written.

ALAN LAMB helped in the editing of the book.

HAZEL, my wife, has always been my personal supporter and public defender, taking up the challenge when needed.

I also owe thanks to my editor/agent, KEN BOHANNON, of The Writer's Advocate, for teaching me about commas and for his help and suggestions, which greatly improved the manuscript.

Last, I owe thanks to MY SPIRITUAL GUIDE, who has steered me through critical times, leading me to focal points of self- and cosmic revelation. He has always been there like a good Zen master to knock me down in brief moments of glory, forcing me to assess and reevaluate my position.

CONDITIONED
REFLEXES

A YOUNG MAN sat in my office for the first time. He had been coming to the clinic for several years, but this was the first time he had seen me. I hefted his chart, which was fully an inch thick.

"And what is your problem, Harry?" I leafed quickly through pages and pages of doctors' notes, X-ray, CT scan and laboratory reports. Every test result was normal.

"It's my migraine headaches. I get them all the time, and they're getting worse. They just hit me on top of the head. I don't have to be doing anything, working or anything, and they hit me right here." He placed his hand on top of his head to show me the spot.

There was nothing in the chart to suggest a true migraine. After I had talked with him, I was certain his head pain did not fit into any recognized pain syndrome. Yet every one of the other doctors had diagnosed it as a migraine. In addition to the scores of normal tests, there were consultations with neurologists, neurosurgeons, ENT men, and psychiatrists. None of the consultants had anything further to offer, beyond repeating tests that had previously been performed and were already known to be negative. No one who had seen Harry had been able to step outside the narrow, constrained thought processes in which they had been conditioned. In the thinking of most doctors, there are only a few causes of headache: migraine, tension, histamine headache, trigeminal neuralgia, eye strain, trauma, and intracranial space-occupying lesions, such as tumors. I can think of five or six additional causes off the top of my mind.

My colleagues were not stupid. They were as fine a group of physicians as one was likely to encounter anywhere. They certainly were not motivated to run all those tests to make money, for in our HMO the more we spent on tests the less we all received at the end of the year in the form of bonuses. They were ordering the tests and consultations in a sincere attempt to diagnose the cause of the headache. They were good guys all, and, except for two or three, I was truly fond of them.

Unfortunately, like most physicians, they were trapped into rigid patterns of thought, belief, and action brought on through years of the intellectual brainwashing that has passed for medical education. Actually, doctors are poorly educated! Their education consists of training along a very narrow path, and they wear huge intellectual blinders as they go. Anything appearing in their intellectual peripheral vision is suspect, frightening, and likely to be ignored.

"Look, Harry, I don't think you have a migraine, and you don't have a brain tumor either. What do you say about letting me hypnotize you to see if we can find out just what's causing your headaches? If you turn out to be a good subject, I think I can help you."

"Sure. Let's give it a whirl," he said, "I'll try anything."

Fortunately, Harry was an excellent subject. In a few minutes, he was in a deep trance. I asked him to go back to the first time his head ever hurt like it did now. I directed him to go to before the pain started so that we could find out just what led up to it. He hesitated a long time and I reinforced the suggestion, telling him his subconscious mind remembered everything and that he should just relax and let the memory come. Finally, he began to smile, relating that he was on his way to visit his girlfriend. He had picked a bouquet of wild flowers and was walking to her house to see her.

Picking a bouquet of flowers seemed a bit unusual—at least in this day and age—so I asked him what year we were talking about. After quite a long pause, he said "1784." I asked where he was living and he told me a short distance from Atlanta. He went on to explain that Atlanta wasn't very big then, more like a large town. He continued to recall old memories. He said that, as he was walking through a patch of woods, he was attacked by four thugs bent on robbing him. Three of them held him while the fourth beat him on top of the head with a club, until his skull was crushed. I continued to question him, looking for the set of circumstances that would trigger the subconscious memories of the pain and murder.

Just as I had suspected, the headaches were nothing more than a response to a conditioned reflex. The trigger that brought on the headache was a complex of several things: a nice day, a feeling of happiness, preparing to have an enjoyable time. I told Harry the episode had occurred about 200 years ago in another life, and to another head. There was nothing wrong with his present head. It had not been injured. I went on to explain—with Harry still under hypnosis—that circumstances of being happy, a pretty day, and planning a good time were not, and never had been, related to the original cause of the head pain. Through the next several years, I saw him for some minor problems, but the headaches never recurred. This one case is a perfect example of a symptom, or an illness, caused by a conditioned reflex. The process is quite common and usually goes unrecognized by the members of the medical profession.

Conditioned reflexes were first described by a Russian physiologist named Ivan Pavlov. In his classic experiment, he placed food in front of a dog and noticed that the sight and smell of the food caused the dog's mouth to water. He proceeded to do this day after day, and at the same time he placed the food in front of the dog, he rang a bell. The dog began to associate the sound of the bell with the food. After a while, Pavlov simply rang the bell and the dog's mouth would begin to water, even though no food was present. This act of salivation triggered by a normally unrelated stimulus is called a conditioned reflex.

Experimentation has shown that there is no body function that cannot be initiated or altered through the process of conditioning. Usually, it takes a number of repeated episodes to establish a reflex, but, if the situation is right, one association is enough to establish a lasting response. Such was the case with Harry. Furthermore, the reflex persisted even though no conditioning had occurred in *Harry's* life. His spiritual memory continued to initiate the reflex within a physical body that had not suffered any attack.

It is important to understand the underlying principle taking place within the body that allows a conditioned reflex to develop, for this principle is central to comprehending not only conditioned reflexes but every aspect of health and disease. Every cell in the body is a separate living unit with qualities of individual consciousness all its own. Cells do not sit passively within the tissue of which they are a part, receiving oxygen and nutrients from the blood as it circulates through the body. Research spanning the Twentieth Century has indicated that each cell is constantly "aware," making decisions and performing its various functions as an individual intelligent unit of life. These decisions are made within the limit of certain constraints and with total cooperation of the tissue or organ in which the cell is located. A muscle cell could not go wandering about or begin to behave as if it were a connective tissue cell. Nor could a white blood cell start contracting and act like a muscle cell. Nonetheless, the cells do select nutrients as they are needed and make other discrete and specific decisions and actions on their own.

The organization of cells within the body could be likened to a community of people who band together in groups called towns and states to form a nation in which each social organization serves a separate and distinct function. In a community as perfect as a human body, each individual would direct his or her intent and actions toward joyful cooperation with the intent of the leaders and for the common good of the entire community. Furthermore, every citizen would be ready to alter his or her function on directions from the governing head. Thus, in times of war, peaceful activities directed toward orderly living would be suspended in order to direct all the energies toward defense.

In the workings of your body, the individual cells use their freedom of choice and intent to cooperate with the other cells composing the tissue or organ so as to carry out the primary directions of that organ or tissue. Underlying this whole society of intent is the cells' knowledge and ability to keep themselves in good health and repair and, when appropriate, to restructure and create new cells to take their place when repairing the damage is no longer possible. This mandate, this Prime Directive—to remain healthy in cell and body—is an extremely powerful, fully vested interest. The ability to accomplish this is due in part to the information coded within the genes and contained within the nucleus of each cell.

Remember, the cells are not mindless automatons following a genetic blueprint, but conscious individual units with sufficient degrees of freedom to make choices on their own. Aside from their own internal guidance and their mandate to remain in perfect health and repair, the cells are constantly receiving instruction from your subconscious mind, which has the power to alter the primary orders. In the situation in which a conditioned reflex is formed, the cells take instruction from the subconscious memory and react according to overriding instructions and information from the subconscious mind. With Harry's headache, every time the proper external conditions were noted, the subconscious mind reminded the cells of Harry's conviction that his skull had once been crushed. The cells joyfully cooperated in producing the pain that went along with the injury and those triggering events of anticipating a nice day and so on.

Other diseases are created in the same way. If, as a child, you are conditioned to believe that going out in chilly weather without your hat and sweater will cause a cold, your cellular consciousness will join certain viruses that are always present within your body to produce the cold according to instructions. The same mechanism produces diseases such as cancer, heart attacks, and nearly all others. If you hold a firm belief and fear that you will develop a cancer as did your mother or father, this belief may eventually take the form of instructions to your cellular consciousness to produce the very cancer you fear. On the other hand, if you picture yourself as healthy and with great powers of resistance to illness and disease, your belief will augment the primary instructions of the cells to remain healthy, and it will be a rare occurrence that you become ill. In short, both health and illness ultimately depend, in large part, upon the internal instructions being given to the cellular consciousness.

I had another headache case which will further illustrate how conditioned reflexes operate and are produced. A twelve-year-old boy in my practice was having increasingly severe tension headaches. Like Harry's, they would come on out of the blue, for no apparent reason. The family was fairly new to me, and, since they were not the type to run to the doctor for minor problems, I had seen him only once before with a headache.

One noon, his father called, saying that Donald had gotten one of his bad headaches when he came home for lunch, and asked if I would see him. I had him bring the boy in. Donald was really hurting, holding his head and almost moaning. His father helped him onto the exam table. I asked Donald if he would let me hypnotize him and take the pain away. He was willing to do anything that would relieve his headache.

Donald went easily into a good trance, and I suggested the pain away. Then I asked him to remember back in time to before his head ever hurt so that we could find out what caused the pain. Immediately, he recalled an episode when he was about four. He was playing with some children when a fight broke out. In the scuffle, Donald was hit in the head with a ball bat. Naturally, he got a headache. I asked him to go to the next time he got a headache. He recalled an incident a couple of years later when he and his sister were having a fight. Somehow, he had tripped, striking his head. A third episode occurred when he was ill with chicken pox. He was running a high fever, had a headache, and his parents were in his bedroom having a heated argument. Hearing these accounts, I pointed out to Donald that there had been a fight or argument on each occasion. Then I suggested he come back to the present and go to the time just before his current headache started.

"I'm way ahead of you, Dr. Bonnett. I came home for lunch and an old cowboy movie was on the TV. The actors started a fight and the headache began. That's funny, the fighting didn't actually have anything to do with my headaches. I guess I really don't have to have them."

"Wow, Donald, you get an A+ in physiology!" I exclaimed. He never experienced another headache.

Shelly was another good example of a conditioned reflex in action. She was terribly allergic to cat dander. On more than one occasion, I had made a house call in the middle of the night to give her a shot of adrenaline to stop an asthma attack after she had been in someone's home who owned a cat. Furthermore, I had done allergy skin tests, and she reacted violently to cat dander. There was no question that she had a true allergy to cats, resulting in asthma attacks.

This was a time in my practice when I was using a lot of hypnosis, so I talked her into letting me hypnotize her to determine what might be accomplished. She agreed. When Shelly was a little girl, her mother had worked, so she was raised by a housekeeper who was obsessive-compulsive, totally concerned with cleanliness. To the housekeeper, a tiny spot of dirt was a catastrophe. At the slightest bit of soil, Shelly's dress would be changed, and she would suffer a long lecture about how terrible it was to get dirty.

Under hypnosis, I asked Shelly to go back in time to just before she ever had trouble breathing. She recalled a day when she was about three, playing with a kitten in a sandbox. When the kitten "mussed" her dress, Shelly ran into the house crying and sobbing. The housekeeper did her usual thing, changing Shelly's dress, while making a big fuss about how terrible it was to get dirty.

"Then what happened?" I asked.

"The doctor's coming."

"Why?"

"Because I'm having an asthma attack."

"Why?"

"Because I'm allergic to cats. You know that," she snapped.

"Come on, Shelly, you weren't having any trouble until the cat peed on your dress. Are you still crying?"

"No."

"I presume you mean the tears have stopped. Are you still sobbing, like this?" I mimicked the sound of wheezing by taking in my breath while constricting my vocal cords.

"Yes."

The doctor arrived. Little Shelly was still making the sobbing noises. He asked what she had been doing and was told only that she had been playing with a kitten. Then, in his infinite wisdom, he announced that Shelly was allergic to cats and was having an asthma attack as a result of playing with the kitten.

A second episode occurred shortly thereafter, when she was playing with some other children. Things weren't going her way, so she decided to cry. She began sobbing, and her mother rushed into the room. A cat just happened to be present, too. Her mother snatched Shelly up, stating she was having an asthma attack caused, of course, by the presence of the cat. There were a couple of other episodes that cemented the conditioned reflex. After that, the cells of her respiratory tract knew exactly what to do when she inhaled cat dander. I pointed out to her—while she was still hypnotized—that the cat was not related to the breathing difficulty except in an associative way. I suggested that she, therefore, didn't need to have asthma anymore. In this instance, as with Harry's headache, I was actually re-instructing her cellular consciousness to return to its primary mode of functioning while, at the same time, telling her subconscious mind to ignore the misinformation that had been given to her by her doctor.

Several weeks later, I was at her home. Shelly reached down and scooped up a fuzzy kitten from beneath the dining room table. She held it up to her face, rubbing her cheek and nose into its fur.

"Look what I have. It was a stray, and so cute I couldn't resist it."

"Gee, I thought you were allergic to cats," I replied.

"Don't be ridiculous," she quipped. "I never was."

She had no more asthma. Once the mechanism of the conditioned reflex is pointed out to the individual involved, the reflex is usually abolished. Hypnosis is an excellent medium through which to do this.

I had one patient, a woman, who suffered from severe reactive hypoglycemia. In other words, when she ate sugar her body reacted by making too much insulin. After an hour or two, her blood sugar would plunge to very low levels and she would often pass out. She was on a diet that eliminated sweets, but she continued to have problems, even when she had not eaten food containing sugar. I tested her with a drink sweetened with an artificial sweetener, telling her it contained sugar. An hour later she was on the verge of passing out. Her blood sugar was tested and found to be only thirty-five. True to her conditioned reflex, she reacted to the *taste* of sweet with the production of excess insulin, just as though the drink had actually contained sugar.

Bykov, working at the Pavlovian Institute of Physiology, reports amazing physiologic changes that have been demonstrated through conditioning. In one experiment, researchers at the institute placed a tube into a dog's stomach and poured in 1500 cc of water. That's about a quart and a half of liquid. Then they measured how much urine the dog produced over the next four hours. The dog's kidneys, with all that extra water in him, did just what yours would do. His kidneys put out a huge volume of very dilute urine in order to get rid of the extra fluid. After doing this every day over the next couple of weeks, putting the tube in the dog's stomach, pouring in the water, and measuring the urine output, the kidney tubules and the dog's mind were conditioned.

Then they put the tube down into the dog's stomach but *did not* pour in any water at all. The dog's kidneys proceeded to make the same volume of dilute urine they had been making every day since the experiment started. The urine was dilute and the volume the same, despite the fact there was no excess water to excrete. In this case, the dog associated the introduction of the stomach tube with the need to produce a lot of urine.

Mary came to me because of a rash that would appear on the front and insides of her thighs. It would appear suddenly and was painful rather than itchy. It looked less like a rash and more like scrapes and scratches, but she denied doing anything that could have scratched her legs.

Under hypnosis, Mary recalled a church picnic she attended as a little girl. She was running and playing with a bunch of kids, and her mother warned her that she would get overly tired and make herself sick. But Mary was having too much fun playing tag and climbing trees to quit. She was wearing shorts and, unnoticed by her, she had scraped her thighs on the tree trunks. Finally, her mother forced her to stop playing. When she observed Mary's scratched legs she scolded her daughter for ignoring her earlier warnings. Fatigue was the trigger, and in Mary's mind, it was associated with scraped legs. Thereafter, every time Mary became tired—doing a big washing, cleaning the house, or working in the yard—her thighs would break out in the "rash." With a hypnotic suggestion that fatigue did not *have* to produce the rash, and in fact had no relation to it, Mary had no more trouble.

Conventional medicine had no solution for any of these cases. If I had been content to stay within the confines of "standard medical care," Harry and Donald would still have their headaches, going from doctor to doctor, specialist to specialist, searching for help. Nothing would have worked, and most likely they would have become hooked on tranquilizers, all the while in constant search of stronger pain medicine. Eventually, because their pain did not fit into any recognized syndrome, they would probably each have ended up with a psychiatrist who would have tried to force them into his belief system, blaming repressed sexual problems and bad parenting for their troubles. Shelly would have been relegated to a life of allergy shots, bronchial dilators, steroids, and perhaps a psychiatrist, too, since asthma is known to have an emotional component. Mary would have ended up smearing on ointments and swallowing antihistamines every time she felt tired.

Without a physician's going beyond conventional medical practice, none of these patients would have been properly diagnosed, nor would the treatments prescribed have been appropriate to address the real causes of their difficulties. Needless to say, their psychotherapy would, more than likely, have been unsuccessful as well.

I think it obvious, just from the cases discussed here, that conditioned reflexes can and do play a major role in the development of some illness. What's more, standard approaches to treatment are often inappropriate and doomed to fail because they do not acknowledge the real dynamics of disease.

Hypnosis is an excellent investigative and therapeutic tool, for, through its use, a doctor can speak more or less directly with the bio-consciousness and the subconscious mind, with little or no interference from the ego. But most doctors are unskilled in its use, and not every patient is capable of attaining an adequately deep trance for effective work. Hypnosis is also time consuming, but when one considers how effective it can be, the time is well spent. Still, the public in general does not accept hypnosis as a proper tool for physicians. They accept it fairly well from psychiatrists, but the idea of the family doctor using it is a bit weird. In my own practice, I had a few patients leave me when it got around that I was using hypnosis. Apparently, they were uncomfortable going to a doctor with such nonstandard procedures.

Doctors must be willing to accept the idea that conditioned reflexes can be responsible for illnesses in their patients, bother to understand the actual mechanism that takes place at the cellular level, and accept that conditioned responses are not just something they read about in medical school. Once this first step of enlightenment takes place, they just may come to understand that hypnosis can help them to diagnose and treat biophysical problems. Or maybe they'll refer their patients to someone who does. The problem is that enlightenment seems unlikely, at least on any broad scale. Far too many physicians are afraid of being nonconformists or are unwilling to go to the trouble of incorporating new ideas into their shared belief system. In a way, that is the fault of the educational system and of the individuals who make up the members of the medical profession.

PROBLEMS WITH DOCTORS

I 'VE SPENT CONSIDERABLE TIME figuring out just how I came to be so different in my approach to medicine and to hold such a radically different view of the nature of humankind from those of my colleagues. To appreciate my differences, it is necessary to know what the average doctor is like and how so many of them got that way. I wish to make it absolutely clear that what I am about to say does not apply to every doctor. But I believe it does apply to the medical profession in general. Thus, when I write "doctors," "physicians" or "the medical profession," I intend the remark to apply generically to doctors and the profession. In all honesty, some observations and characteristics probably apply to me as well. Certainly, I was not totally immune to the brainwashing of the educational system through which beliefs, ideas, concepts, and prejudices are engraved into the minds of most every individual who attends a medical school. The only thing that saved me was that, somewhere inside, a small portion of my mind refused to accept the lesson completely. I owe this to my parents.

As a child, I was totally accepted as an important, valuable individual and a full, equal member of the family. We used to talk about everything. In fact, some years ago, when my father was dying of pneumonia, I confessed to him that I could not think of anything to visit about at the moment. He laughed, saying we had talked about every possible subject all our lives and there was no way there could be anything left to say. I had to agree with him, so I told him again that I loved him and held his hand while he died.

The point I want to make is that I was raised in a loving, supportive relationship. I can never remember, even once, being told that the topic under discussion was none of my affair or to be quiet because I didn't know what I was talking about. My folks listened to what I had to say. My input was accepted, and when I was not being logical or reasonable, we discussed my viewpoint. Skillfully, they guided my thinking without putting me down. They were wise, too, and that helped. In this supportive atmosphere, I grew up trusting them and holding a clear view that my thoughts and ideas were valid.

In addition, my father was a world-renowned scientist in the field of plant genetics and morphology. He wrote a number of papers on the morphologic development of wheat, oats, barley, and corn. His work on the development of the corn plant won him a Guggenheim Fellowship in 1947. Two concepts my father handed down to me were a conviction to finish every project and the love of searching for new ways to do things. If a tried-and-true method exists that is 70 percent effective, perhaps another could be found that is 95 percent effective. He taught me that it is worth the try, for, unless a search is made for something better, one will always be stuck with a method only 70 percent effective. If you are unsuccessful, you can always fall back on the old way. Nothing will be lost in the attempt. Hence, I was always interested in trying new approaches in medicine, especially when the standard treatments were only marginally successful.

When it came to trying different things, I always did it with enthusiasm and zeal. If one is truly interested in attempting experimentation, the honest way is to give it the best shot. If one hangs back, halfheartedly involved, even an excellent plan may fail. While proceeding to explore a new idea in my practice, I was constantly monitoring the process and the results in the back of my mind. After a fair trial, I would evaluate the total situation to determine whether to drop the idea or continue. Most of my colleagues never understood what I was doing, nor did they appreciate the monitoring process taking place. Instead, they perceived me as "forever going off on some kick."

It is my experience that too few individuals go into medicine with the primary goal of helping people. If you can get them to admit it, all too many doctors chose the medical profession, first and foremost, to get rich. But medicine is a poor vehicle to wealth. The training process is too long, and the work hours are excessive. Other ways to make money are a lot easier, if that is your goal.

When I first started practice, I was visiting with my uncle, who was a physician. He taught me that a doctor is responsible for the patients he sees, not for all the patients who would like to see him. He went on to say that I should, therefore, be content with the income those patients would generate. If money is one's goal, there is always more to be made. Upon coming out of retirement to do a special show, Jack Benny was once asked why with all his money he had gone to work again. Benny quipped, "I found out I didn't have it all." As my practice developed, I came to appreciate fully my uncle's wisdom. Too many doctors crowd their schedules with so many patients that they can't properly diagnose or treat any of them.

To some extent, doctors are attracted to medicine because it is interesting and exciting. Like most folks, we read books and watch movies and TV programs about doctors, and we often end up confusing fiction with reality. Unfortunately, for some, the God-like power that accompanies medicine is appealing. The aura of omnipotence surrounding medicine is as addicting as the desire for money. These goals are actually, albeit unwittingly, cultivated and nurtured by the educational system. The system doesn't set out to produce greedy gods; such doctors are just a by-product.

So we have a lot of young people heading into the medical profession for a lot of different reasons, some of which are not very healthy. One thing is certain, the reasons don't contribute to the production of the kind of doctor most people want or think they have.

By the time the doctor starts to practice, he or she may well have developed into what William Philpott calls a poorly educated, slow learner. Dr. Philpott was trained as an analytical psychiatrist. He once told how he became interested in ecologically induced diseases. He said he had been practicing psychiatry for twelve years when he was forced to admit to himself that he had never cured a single psychotic patient. Furthermore, he did not know of any other psychiatrist who had, either. He hadn't even *heard* of a patient being cured. What he had done was to help patients cope with their illnesses. He had successfully talked a few neurotics out of their neuroses, he said, but he had never talked a single patient out of being schizophrenic, depressed, or psychotic.

So Dr. Philpott had quit standard therapy and adopted a new approach that did work. (The method will be discussed later in the book.) In doing so, he met with a lot of resistance. He was supposed to cure people by talking to them or he wasn't supposed to do it at all. Dr. Philpott came to the conclusion that physicians were slow learners, conditioned to be so by their education and belief system. Much of what follows in the next pages are his concepts, which I have expanded based upon my own experience.

Look at the educational system. First of all, grades are of utmost importance. Through high school, premedicine, and medical school, the majority of doctors spend most of their time memorizing tons of material. The curriculum is composed almost exclusively of science subjects, which further contributes to a lack of a broad education. For most med and premed students, studying to make top grades is the primary time-consuming activity.

I was not unusual. In my premedical years, my advisor refused to allow me to take any courses other than the bare essentials. He stressed the importance of having a straight A average to ensure my getting into medical school. So that is what I did. During my four years of medical school, this was a typical day: My alarm would go off at 6:30 in the morning. I would shave, dress, eat breakfast, and be in class at 8:00. Classes would continue until 5:00 in the afternoon. The noon hour consisted of busing tables in exchange for my noon meal. After my evening meal, I would hit the books by 6:30 and continue studying until midnight. Then, I would take a break and go out to the White Castle hamburger stand around the corner for a burger, fries, and a shake. After my break, I'd continue to study until I fell asleep at my desk, usually sometime around 2:00 in the morning. Saturdays were usually spent studying, as were Sunday afternoons and evenings. Once in a great while, I would go to a movie. In those days, I went to church, so Sunday mornings were my only regular break from the grind. It came to the point that I was so exhausted I could not stay awake. Then, like a lot of my classmates, I began studying standing up, placing my books on the top of a chest of drawers. This worked fairly well until I learned one can sleep for hours standing up.

The University of Illinois medical school had a policy in those days of grading on a curve. It didn't matter how well the students did. The grades were adjusted so that 10 percent were flunked on every test, and an equal number were failed every year. On the pharmacology mid-term exam, as I recall, the lowest grade had been a 78. The department head, who was new to the school, angrily confessed to the class that he had been forced to lower the grades in order to fail sixteen students. (As I recall, my grade had been lowered from an 83 to a 76.) He told us he refused to continue teaching at such an institution, and, true to his word, he resigned at the end of the term. The stress was unbelievable.

Knowing what I do now, I would have chosen a different medical school or gone into chiropractic. This kind of system is not interested in education as a primary goal. It resembles more a game of "Gotcha."

During the year of my internship, I was lucky to get three hours' sleep a night. This was often interrupted by telephone calls, trips to restart intravenous fluids, and emergencies. Residency training was somewhat more relaxed. Still, one was on duty twenty-four hours a day, with perhaps a few hours off every week or two. In recent years, the system has changed. Interns and residents these days have more regular hours, free time, and vacations. But despite these changes, the system leaves precious little time for normal socialization.

The years from ages seventeen to about twenty-seven are the important formative years in the development of adult interpersonal skills. During this entire time, future doctors have their heads buried in books. These ten years are the time during which they should have the opportunity to learn to relate to others and to be human beings. But whatever socialization occurs in their lives is mostly with other medical people who are as narrow and poorly socialized as they. The doctors finally graduate and finish training knowing a great deal of factual scientific knowledge but with little real skill in applying it in life situations, for they have been trained not to get close to or familiar with their patients. Highly trained as they may be, they are virtually isolated from feelings, the humanity of their patients, and the world in general. Many new doctors are, therefore, both frightened and defensive.

As a result of this relative isolation from the real world, doctors use huge blocks of medical knowledge as a socialization tool. They utilize it as a means of relating to the world. They converse with their peers—largely about medicine—trying to impress with their vast stores of information and up-to-date knowledge of the latest research. They are driven to read medical journals and are subtly pressured to read the ones in vogue at the time. Doctors may use their knowledge to keep others at arm's length. They may cover themselves with it like armor to insulate themselves from society, while at the same time expecting the non-medical world to be dazzled by the glitter of their knowledge. They insist upon being called "doctor." Too many of them feel superior to others and expect to be granted all sorts of privileges.

The average physician is a lonely, frightened, pathetic, self-serving, insecure, egotistical individual who spends life protecting a holy body of knowledge. Doctors' only security lies in the belief that what they were taught was correct and that they hold the *only* valid system of medical thought, belief, and practice.

When they take courses in continuing education, they largely hear what they already know. In other words, the belief that conventional knowledge is absolutely valid and complete is reinforced. Any new material which may be introduced is only marginally different from what is already known and considered true. The "new" material *must* be securely anchored to what is already accepted as standard. If it is totally new or, still worse, in opposition to what is previously believed, doctors likely never hear about it in the first place, or they reject it out of hand.

Physicians have a vested interest in rejecting new ideas. Part of the reason for this is that most doctors have little training in deductive thinking. What serves as thought is mostly recalling, with accuracy, what has been previously memorized. Medical education consists largely of rote memorization of piles and piles of information. In most classroom situations, all the students are required to do is to remember what they have read or were told, and then apply it to a given situation in an accepted fashion.

Just to illustrate that this statement is not overwrought, let me recount a chilling event from the time of my own education. As we were told the story in medical school, the university had for years done IQ tests on the graduating seniors. The purpose was to see how well the intelligence quotient of the students correlated with their standing in the class. Were the students with the highest IQs tops in the class? Was there any correlation at all? We heard that, a couple of years before we started school, something happened which caused the university to abandon the study. It seems one senior student was about to graduate from medical school with an IQ of a moron. What's more, he was not at the bottom of the class! They analyzed how this could happen and came to the following conclusions. First, he was good at memorization and studied very hard. Second, he was a nice looking, personable young man who tended to stay in the background and not volunteer in class, thereby exposing his lack of intelligence. The real shocker was that the professors, on further examination of the system, had to admit that nowhere in the curriculum were students actually required to think. They concluded that, since he had made passing grades, they couldn't very well prevent him from graduating. Needless to say, they stopped testing IQs.

I once knew a physician who had an emotional breakdown. He was hospitalized and, during the course of the workup, was found to have an IQ of 65. Apparently, he was burned out on booze and barbiturates and suffered chronic brain damage. It was anyone's guess how many years he had been practicing in this mentally deficient state. He was the only doctor in the small town outside Champaign, Illinois, where he practiced. Insofar as we could tell, the patients had not suffered because of his condition. The lesson to be learned from all this is that a sharp intellect is not an absolute requirement to practice acceptable standard medicine—just rote memory and the ability to apply that information in the right situations. He was able to function taking care of simple ordinary illnesses and complaints. Combine this with the fact that most people who see the doctor on any given day don't really require medical assistance in the first place—then everyone lucked out.

Doctors' thought processes are often so compartmentalized that, at times, when there are common factors within different situations, it is next to impossible for them to see the connection. For example, in the preceding chapter with Shelly's allergy to cats, her physician had learned about conditioned reflexes in medical school when he studied physiology. He learned about them in the context of Pavlov's dog and bell. But he failed to apply this to a little girl with a dirty dress, a cat, and an obsessive-compulsive baby-sitter. In his mind, there was no connection. It probably never even occurred to him. He knew of conditioned reflexes in the context of dogs and bells. Cats and kids are something different. When he heard the crowing noise as Shelly continued to fake her crying, it could mean only one thing. In his training, noisy breathing meant asthma. What else could it be? People are often allergic to cats, and allergies lead to asthma. After all, he had been astute enough to inquire what she had been doing prior to the episode. He added it all up and made his diagnosis. He was probably quite proud of his clever detective work.

One of the most compelling reasons physicians reject new ideas is fear of change and the need to protect their block of medical information, which serves as their clearest bridge to others and the world. This block of medical knowledge constitutes an area of intellectual territory. Humans, like all creatures, are territorial. Studies show that obtaining and holding a territory is *the* primary basic drive. Even the sex drive is secondary to maintaining a territory. Think about it. What good is accomplished by breeding if there is no territory in which to raise the young? Territory ensures shelter, food, safety, and protection from competition. We are all territorial. If you don't believe it, imagine what would happen if your neighbor started parking his car in your driveway or, worse still, built his fence on your property.

With most professionals, knowledge is regarded as territory. But I know of no other profession that guards it quite as jealously as do physicians. To the doctor, it is absolutely critical. New ideas constitute a threat to the territory. To accept a new concept as valid implies that somewhere inside this sacred mass of knowledge lies a thought that is untrue or obsolete. Once a doctor allows that possibility to exist—the possibility that some medical knowledge is inaccurate or obsolete—then potentially there is no end to the changes in belief structure that might be required. Being afraid to cope with this potential intellectual chaos, doctors tend to reject new ideas. Incidentally, most people can't handle the concept of two seemingly opposite facts existing within the same belief construct at the same time. Truths do not negate one another. If they appear to do so, then only two possibilities exist. The one is that an unperceived, underlying truth has created an apparent contradiction. The other possibility is that one or both "truths" are, in fact, untrue. In either case, when doctors are confronted with ideas that do not fit into their belief systems, it is easier and safer, from their perspective, to reject them.

New—really new—material is rarely presented at medical lectures nor often found in "accepted" medical literature. Editors simply refuse to print it, and the lecturers, who are steeped in conventional wisdom, have, therefore, probably never heard of it. Editors fear the possibility that new material may in the future be proved inaccurate and that they will, thus, find themselves subject to ridicule. I heard one editor of a medical journal state during a forum on medical education that doctors, being extremely busy, cannot afford to take time to think. What's more, he felt doctors were incapable of making valid judgments concerning new information. His position, as well as that of the others on the forum, was that the tired, over-worked physician needs to pick up a journal and read feeling secure that what he or she reads is standard and accepted. Again, the system reinforces the doctors' belief that their knowledge is complete. It reminds me of an old saying: It takes fifty years to get a new idea into the medical literature, and 200 years to get the inaccurate and obsolete things removed.

What all this does is keep the truly brilliant thinkers and those physicians and scientists who are actually leading in their fields on the fringes of their professions. They are branded nonconformists and therefore treated with mistrust and ridicule. Being considered a nonconformist—even worse than a malpractice suit—is the greatest fear facing a doctor who might otherwise be tempted to try some alternative approach to a problem. The results of unorthodox treatment or scientific research, no matter how successful or well performed, are almost always rejected by the editorial boards of the medical journals. In order to get their work into print, the noncon- formists turn to writing books. But even if the books are read by their peers, the information is usually discounted because an editorial board did not pass judgment upon it and make certain it was well anchored in standard, accepted medical knowledge. So we are back to square one in a perfect "Catch 22." Linus Pauling once suggested to me over lunch that medical schools needed a department of theo- retical medicine, just as there are departments of theoretical mathe- matics and physics. The establishment of a department of theoretical medicine would go a long way in loosening up the rigid thought pat- terns of the teaching institutions. Let a group of free-thinking doc- tors make some theoretical statements about how things ought to work and what alternate treatments might be useful. Then let others go about the task of proving or disproving the ideas.

In all fairness to the medical profession, it is not the only one behaving in such a fashion. All professions do, to one degree or another. Let me digress with an interesting story. One day, a gradu- ate student came to my father for advice. It seemed he was unable to get the research paper published on which he had received his Ph.D. He had submitted it to numerous agricultural and botanical jour- nals, but they had all refused to publish it. Dad read the paper and asked what the problem was, since it appeared to be well written and an excellent piece of scientific work.

The research involved submitting soybean seed to a large amount of radiation in an effort to produce mutations. The student had given seed the quantity of X-ray the literature said should be enough to produce mutations. But no mutations had appeared when he grew the seed. Finally, in desperation, he gave some more seed a huge dose—so huge, in fact, that it should have sterilized the seed. Truth was, most of the seeds were killed, but the few beans that did germinate produced very interesting mutations. A good experiment. The reason the editors gave for rejecting the paper was that they

didn't believe him. They insisted his research was flawed. They assert-
ed that *all* the seed should have been sterilized. Therefore, he could
not have given the amount of radiation he claimed he had.

My father told him that if he wanted his paper published, he
should submit it to a physics journal. Dad reasoned that the physi-
cists would not be prejudiced against the paper since they wouldn't
be as familiar with the dose of X-ray supposedly lethal to soybean
seed. The student sent his paper to one of the leading physics journals where it was not only accepted, but became the lead article in
the next issue. So much for rigidity.

The medical profession is so cloistered in its position that
information which does not corroborate what has already appeared
in medical literature tends to be considered invalid or, at best, is not
fully trusted. This is true no matter how prestigious the journal may
be. Certainly, there are scores of scientific journals whose standards
are at least as high as, or higher than, for that matter, any medical
journal's. When a person takes it upon himself to write an article for
a medical journal, his head doesn't suddenly open up so God can
pour in wisdom and knowledge. On occasion, when I made some
statement of fact not generally known by my colleagues, I would be
questioned as to my source of information. If I replied I had read it
in a journal such as *Science* or the *Journal of Experimental Biology and
Medicine,* I would invariably be met with sneers of disbelief. It did not
count if the information was not found in the *New England Journal of
Medicine* or some other source commonly accepted and read by
physicians. Speaking of arrogance, one medical school professor
who was a physician once made the statement that every professor
on the faculty who was not a physician should be dropped from the
staff. It was his opinion that only a physician was qualified to instruct
another physician.

Example could be piled upon example illustrating the rigid
mind-set of the medical profession. At one time, I became intensely
interested in the motor-perceptual development of children. The

physicians in Champaign-Urbana were threatened by my doing something they did not understand. I was applying new-found knowledge—at least new to the medical world—and getting good results. According to conventional wisdom, what was happening was impossible. The ophthalmologists banded together and tried unsuccessfully to discipline me and force me out of the county medical society.

During this stressful time, I read *The Cry and the Covenant,* by Sinclair Lewis, a historical novel based on the life of Ignaz Semmelweis. Prior to the discovery of bacteria, Semmelweis proved childbirth infections were due to bits of dead tissue from the bodies of women who had died of the infection. Of course, the dead tissue and pus were laden with disease germs. Those were the days before rubber gloves and the germ theory of disease. Doctors would do an autopsy on a woman who had died of a childbirth infection, wipe their bloody, pus-covered hands on the lapels of their frock coats, and then do a vaginal exam on a woman in labor. Naturally, that woman became infected and died of childbed fever, too.

Semmelweis discovered that by washing his hands in phenol and not doing pelvic exams he could prevent the disease from spreading throughout his obstetrical ward. While the other doctors were experiencing death rates as high as 60 or 70 percent, Semmelweis reduced the death rate on his ward to almost zero.

The doctors were jealous and probably frightened. Besides, this new concept was foreign to their belief system. Epidemics were thought to be due to bad air hanging over a city and other things of this kind. Imagine! The idea that they were spreading the disease! After all, they were doctors! Rather than trying Semmelweis's procedures themselves, they would sneak onto his ward in the dead of night and do vaginal exams on his patients with their filthy hands. The nurses and patients were threatened in order to keep them silent. Of course, there was an outbreak of infections on Semmelweis's ward and many women and babies died. Afterward, the other doctors jeered at him, asking what had gone wrong with his theory. It took Semmelweis quite a while to discover what was taking place. Reading the book, I became physically ill and had to put it aside for a time. I realized the medical profession, which the public holds in such high regard, has not changed all that much.

When I first started practice, I looked about at the other physicians in the community. I was sickened by what often took place. Many, not all, but many of the doctors seemed to have little regard for their patients as persons. While making every effort to ensure the patients were getting well, they also did what was most expedient (or what would give them the largest income). Doctors want their patients to recover, for this reflects on their ability as physicians, and a good reputation is necessary to garner a big practice. Increasing income, sometimes termed "working one's practice," ranges from unnecessary injections of medicine just as effectively administered by mouth to "churning" their practice. Churning is the practice of having patients return more frequently than necessary, thereby producing more income for the doctor. One doctor I knew would give a woman with a vaginal yeast infection a prescription for medicine he knew was totally inappropriate. Several days later, she would return even worse than before. If she was not complaining too badly he would change to a medicine equally ineffective. On about her third trip, he would prescribe the proper vaginal cream. This practice gave him two extra office calls when he could have treated the lady with the correct medicine the first time. It cost the poor woman a lot of money for useless medicine and office calls, not to mention an extra week or two of suffering.

Some doctors I knew in those days dispensed medicine from their office rather than writing prescriptions. The medicine was invariably cheap and often obsolete. But it could be purchased for pennies and sold to the patients at great profit.

Surgery was often performed for minor indications and the true facts distorted out of proportion when the surgeon wrote the hospital record. This made the patient's symptoms appear far worse than they really were. The surgery, if one believed the hospital record, appeared justified when the surgical case review committee reviewed the chart. Several examples of surgical dishonesty I encountered deserve telling.

The wife of a man I had known almost all my life came to me as a new patient. She wanted a physical because she was tired and weak, and she was concerned about the very heavy menstrual periods she was having. As a part of the history, I inquired about any previous surgery she might have had. She gave me this list of five separate operations performed upon her:

1. Appendectomy
2. Removal of the left ovary and tube
3. Removal of her entire uterus
4. Removal of a cyst from her right ovary
5. Removal of the right ovary and tube

These operations had been done by a doctor in Danville, a town about thirty miles away, over a period of seven or eight years. Now, a woman with no pelvic organs in her body doesn't have anything to produce a menstrual period. On physical exam, she had a huge mass in her lower abdomen extending above her navel. The pelvic examination revealed her cervix to be present, and so was a huge fibroid uterus. Running down the midline of her lower abdomen were several scars. She was 52 years old and anemic from the excessive vaginal bleeding, so I recommended a hysterectomy.

At surgery, except for the scars on her lower abdomen, there was no evidence of the surgeon's ever having been in her belly. Nothing had been removed. She still had her uterus, both ovaries, and tubes, as well as her appendix. This trusting lady had undergone five separate operations and general anesthetics, with only a bunch of scars to show for the risks she had taken.

Another case involved the wife of a young bank officer whom I had seen on several occasions with a gallbladder attack. Her gallbladder was full of stones, and I had advised her to have it out. She decided to delay the surgery until after their vacation. About a month after she returned, she came to the office saying she had gotten sick on vacation and had her gallbladder removed by a surgeon in Michigan. But she was experiencing a recurrence of her right upper-quadrant pain. I explained to her and her husband that a stone in the bile duct might have been missed, through no fault of the surgeon. I ordered some X-rays designed to demonstrate gall duct stones. To my surprise, there was her gallbladder, full of stones, just as it had been before. Needless to say, the patient and her husband could hardly believe it, for the surgeon had shown "her" gallbladder to her and given her a couple of "her" stones. I operated and removed her gallbladder. Except for the scar, there was no evidence the other surgeon had done anything whatsoever.

These two cases are flagrant examples of patients' being exposed to all the risks of anesthetic and surgery, plus the expense, for no purpose other than greed on the part of the doctors, who may have been incapable of performing the appropriate operations. The next case I will relate involves a surgeon, an anesthetist, and a hospital covering themselves by falsifying an entire hospital record. The case involved my wife's best friend, Clara.

Clara was visiting in our home and was lying on the sofa one evening. For no reason other than that she had a long history of high blood pressure, I examined her feet for arterial pulses. There were none, and her feet were cold to the touch. I examined the back of her knees for the pulse in the popliteal artery—none there either. With her permission, I tried to find a pulse in the femoral arteries located in the crease of her groins. Neither artery had a pulse. I asked if her legs cramped when she walked. She replied she could walk only fifty feet or so before having to stop and rest her legs. The woman had almost no circulation in either leg. At my urging she consulted a vascular surgeon when she returned home. Arteriograms revealed both common iliac arteries were totally blocked. The only blood going to either leg was through some collateral vessels. She needed grafts from the aorta to the femoral arteries of both legs.

The surgeon scheduled and performed the surgery. From the standpoint of the grafts, he did a good job. He saved her legs. The problem was she sustained a cardiac arrest on the operating table. Clara was in the operating room about seven or eight hours. When the surgeon finally talked to her husband, he said her heart had stopped and they had experienced a lot of trouble starting it again. When she finally woke up from the anesthetic, it was obvious that Clara was brain damaged. She had no short-term memory. Eventually, she was discharged from the hospital. As the years passed, she became steadily worse.

About a year later, she asked me to prescribe medicine for her blood pressure, since her doctor seemed unable to bring it down to normal. I agreed and requested she have her hospital record sent to me so I could see the EKGs taken before and after her cardiac arrest.

When I received the copy of the hospital chart, it contained everything—the history and physical, anesthetic record, the surgeon's operative record, the recovery room record, nurses' notes, the works—everything except two records. There were no EKGs, and nowhere was there any mention of her heart stopping! The anesthetic record showed a normal pulse and blood pressure throughout the procedure. The surgeon had not mentioned one word about the arrest in the dictation of the operative procedure. Nothing! The whole record had been rewritten—faked! During the time of an emergency, nurses chart things as they occur. The charting isn't always complete as procedures are done, but notes are made and these become included in the permanent record at the time charting is completed. There was no reason to get together and make a pact among all the people involved before the operation was begun. I can only assume the chart was rewritten in the medical record library by the head medical record librarian, the hospital administrator, the surgeon and his assistant, the anesthetist, the operating room supervisor, the recovery room supervisor, and the director of nurses.

All that work and conspiracy were unnecessary. Our friends were not about to sue anyone. Clara had been the head of the hospital's credit department for thirty years. She and her husband understood that doctors and hospitals are not infallible. I have seen hospital records altered in my long years of practice. I have never done it myself, but it is done. This is the most flagrant case I have ever heard of.

Other, less dramatic examples of unethical conduct added to my disenchantment with medicine as practiced by physicians who were supposed to be my peers. These, combined with the medical profession's adherence to methods of treatment that historically had never been effective, added to my disillusionment and directed me toward nonconformity. Actually, my bubble of naiveté burst my first year of practice.

Many of you, no doubt, feel I am too harsh. After all, look at the marvelous advances the profession has accomplished. Look, for instance, at how much longer people are living today.

Let us examine the facts. Take, for example, the life expectancy of white males born in the year 1850 compared with those born in 1986. In 1850, a white baby boy had a life expectancy of 38.3 years. In 1986—136 years later—the life expectancy was 72 years. Obviously quite a change. However, in 1850, those men who had attained the age of 70 years could expect to live another 10.2 years. Now here is the interesting part, a real kicker. In 1986, a 70-year-old man could look forward to 11.7 years more. That's only one and a half years longer! In other words, in 1850 if a child survived the ravages of small pox, measles, infant diarrhea, cholera, and the like, and didn't break a leg and get gangrene, he lived almost as long as his counterpart in 1986. The statistics have changed a bit in recent years, but not much.

No one can say the medical profession has not played a part, but here is a question to ponder: How many millions of dollars are spent keeping those seventy-year-old men alive an average of another eighteen months? Ninety percent of all the money spent on health care in the United States is spent in the last year of the person's life. That's obscene. How much do you want to spend in order for you or Uncle Charlie to have another hour or twelve hours or twelve days or even eighteen months of life? Come on, what is so important to be done that any one of us can't die today? People do it all the time. I'm not advocating refusing treatment to old people who become ill. What I am suggesting is that we must begin to look at all aspects of life, death, and health care and begin to use some judgment.

Most of the gain in longevity has been made not by doctors passing out pills or doing surgery but through public health measures such a vaccines, sewage disposal, water purification, and general sanitation. When I see ads on television showing the wretched conditions in some Third World country, along with a plea from some wealthy actress to give money for relief, I can't help thinking that most of the problems could be solved by the people themselves at little cost. Drinking water can be boiled. People need not throw garbage and sewage into the street. The pigs can be put into pens and the children do not have to play in manure and filth. This is a matter of education, a little work, and a desire to change. It doesn't require money, medicine, or doctors. Much of the problem of the Third World is not so much poverty or lack of food as it is overpopulation. Through allowing custom, indolence, religious beliefs, and lack of birth control to rule over common sense, *the world is breeding itself into extinction.*

How about some of the rich actresses starting to push family planning?

One of the answers is that our holier-than-thou, self-righteous government refused for years to fund family planning here and in other countries.

Ordinary rats have a highly developed social system that prevents overcrowding, maintains proper etiquette while mating, and ensures a safe place for the young to be raised. If the nest is disturbed, the mother rat moves the babies to a safe place. When the population in a given location reaches a critical level, rats simply move away and start another colony where there is adequate space.

An experiment was done in which three large areas were constructed where rats were able to live undisturbed. The pens were built side by side, with walls and electric fences separating the sections. Ladders were present so the rats could distribute themselves equally among the three sections of the enclosure. After the colonies were stable and the rats had evenly distributed themselves, the ladders were removed and an electric fence on top of the dividers was activated. In the middle section, as normal breeding produced overcrowding, rats were removed so the population density was maintained at an acceptable level. The two end sections were allowed to go undisturbed. As population density became a serious problem in the end sections, the rats began to abandon their social courtesies. The male rat ordinarily bites the female gently on the back of the neck during intercourse. The males in the crowded sections sometimes bit the female to death. Young male rats ran in gangs, attacking and attempting to breed with any rat they could catch, young or old, even other males. When the nests were disturbed, female rats would start to move their babies and sometimes drop them on the floor, abandoning them to be eaten by the other rats. Fights occurred constantly. The social environment produced by the overcrowding is termed a "psychological sink."

An interesting development occurred when the ladders were replaced between the end cages where the "sinks" had evolved and the middle section where the normal population density had been maintained. Big, dominant male rats from the normal middle section patrolled the walls and the ladders, keeping the other rats from invading their territory.

In some ways, this illustrates many of the social and behavioral problems seen in areas of the world where overpopulation has become an issue, for whatever the cause or reason. It certainly is something to think about.

In many ways, the world of medicine has changed a lot. In the old days, a patient could tell the doctor to do everything possible. Most of you can't remember back as far as 1925, the year I was born. In those days, there just weren't many specific drugs. Doctors had digitalis for heart failure, morphine for pain, iodine to help loosen chest congestion, aspirin, and not much else. Most medical treatment prescribed by the doctor consisted of various nursing procedures. I can remember the doctor coming to the house when I was sick with a middle ear infection. He would make wise pronouncements like, "Now, we have to keep a close eye on this. We don't want Orville to get a mastoid, or a brain abscess." But there wasn't a blamed thing he could do to prevent it. In those days, if you became ill you got well on your own or died, and the doctor was essentially powerless to affect the course of the illness one way or the other. Nowadays, if you told the doctor to do everything, and if you survived all the tests, you couldn't afford to pay the bill.

Years ago, about 1950, I heard a radio program concerning health care in the United States. A couple of deans of medical schools were on the program. As I recall, one was the dean of Loyola University medical school. Anyway, one of them stated that medical care in this country had reached a point where the diagnostic and therapeutic capabilities staggered the imagination. Imagine, this was 1950! He went on to say that this was one of the best countries in which to become ill if you had a rare or obscure disease. On the other hand, he felt it was one of the worst places to be if you had a simple, minor ailment. His reasoning was that the public had demanded—and the medical profession had gone along with it—that all the tests and treatment modalities designed for use in major illnesses be applied in every minor situation. He went on to relate that if a person chose to see a doctor for a cold, he was likely to receive a chest X-ray, a blood count, and prescriptions for expensive antibiotics. During the last forty-some years, it hasn't gotten any better. The tests are just more expensive, and there are a lot more of them to run.

What I am disturbed about is the narrow focus of medical technology and research. Within the rigid constraints in which the medical profession has worked through the years, tremendous technical advances have been made. Improvement in surgical techniques is unbelievable. Diagnostic instrumentation and equipment approach science fiction. CT scans, nuclear magnetic resonance imagery, the ability to splice chromosomes, all are commonplace. And the list goes on almost indefinitely.

A sick patient is analyzed—by running tests, taking pictures, or whatever—to discover the patho-physiologic changes present in the patient's specific disease. Then the doctor begins adjusting all the little knobs, attempting to tune the body, this organic piece of supposed machinery, back to normal only to find the method doesn't work very well. Then, while the doctor is busy turning knobs, research has discovered another whole set of dials and switches controlling the first set of knobs. The process is endless. The compartmentalization of medical thinking is appalling. Creativity, whether it is in art, writing, or healing a patient cannot be compartmentalized. If the physician is to be a true healer, he or she must cast aside barriers and ideally include input from all directions and healing professions.

I have always felt we should have been looking in the opposite direction. We should have equal enthusiasm for what causes an alteration in normal physiology in the first place. On the surface at least, it appears it would be easier and more cost-effective to keep folks well than to spend untold millions trying to cure them when they are ill—to say nothing of the suffering and lost time at work.

In one of his dialogues, Plato spoke of a physician who was chronically ill. He had managed to stay alive for years by devoting all his time to himself. As Plato phrased it, he kept himself in a constant state of dying. The philosopher went on to say that the common man would not accept this—nor could he afford it. He would, instead, demand the physician cure him or let him die. Not a bad philosophy.

ECOLOGICALLY INDUCED DISEASE

Maladaptive Food Reactions

H UMANKIND IS SUBJECT to a host of illnesses that are a direct result of repeated exposure to elements within the environment. To be certain, toxic chemicals, insect sprays, and industrial wastes have severe effects on public health, but the conditions to which I refer are far more common.

Probably every adult has some illness or symptom which is a direct result of what he or she daily eats, drinks, or breathes. The illnesses include major diseases for which the medical profession has yet officially to determine the cause and can offer no definitive treatment, much less a cure. A partial list of these diseases includes eczema, adult onset diabetes, ulcerative colitis, multiple sclerosis, myasthenia gravis, amyotrophic lateral sclerosis (Lou Gehrig's disease), some forms of muscular dystrophy, schizophrenia, endogenous depression, hyperactivity, rheumatoid arthritis, psoriasis, recurrent thrombophlebitis, chronic bronchitis, asthma, chronic sinusitis, middle-ear effusions, migraine headaches, and others. In addition to these diseases, almost any symptom can be caused by a reaction to what we regularly take into our bodies.

Many less dramatic diseases are also caused by ecological factors. Often, the conditions are so mild and have been present so long that the individual has come to accept them as part of life. Common problems such as fatigue, constipation, post-nasal drip, and chronic acne are so often a part of one's nature that they may be totally overlooked, even on a thorough physical exam. It is important to understand how these illnesses develop and how they may be arrested—sometimes without consulting a physician.

To comprehend maladaptive food reactions, it is necessary to know something about chronic reactions to stress. Dr. Hans Selye, working at the University of Montreal in the 1940s, observed that ill people often seem to have many of the same symptoms, regardless of what is wrong with them. His patients commonly had a low grade fever, ached, were tired, and just didn't feel well. He called this group of symptoms the syndrome of "just being sick."

Later, in his laboratory, he gave groups of white rats daily injections of various substances. It turned out that it didn't really matter much what was injected, for the rats responded to the stress of being captured and stuck with a needle. As a result of the stress, they all developed many of the same symptoms: stomach ulcers, hemorrhages, and infections.

Ultimately, Selye described three phases in the reaction to non-specific acute and chronic stress. The first reaction to stress he called the alarm reaction. The animals appeared to be upset, they didn't eat well, etc. As the stress continued, they began to adjust. They didn't seem to be as disturbed by being captured and stuck with the needle. He called this the stage of adaptation. The third stage began when the adaptive mechanisms started to fail. The animals began to die suddenly with stomach ulcers, hemorrhages, and infections. This phase he named the stage of exhaustion of the adaptive mechanisms, or just "exhaustion" for short.

The body, whether it belongs to a rat or a person, is equipped to make incredible adjustments to change. The problem is that the physiology is not designed to continue these adjustments over long periods of time. Physiologic adaptations wear out after a while. In this respect, your body is a lot like the engine of your automobile. It can operate at extreme speeds for relatively short periods of time, but continued use at excessive speed will wear the engine out more quickly, causing it to break down. This is also true of most, if not all, physiologic processes. As the adaptive mechanisms start to fail, symptoms reappear and diseases become recognized.

Just to make sure you understand how stress disease develops, assume you have a bunch of white rats and have placed them in a room at freezing temperatures in individual cages so they can't huddle together to keep warm. This is too cold for rats, and a certain number will, very shortly, die from exposure to the cold. This collapse of the body physiology from the effects of the cold is the alarm reaction. The cells and metabolism of those rats that don't die will begin to adapt to the environment. They will do so by eating more, so that their basal metabolic rate increases to offset the loss of body heat, their fur grows thicker, etc. In other words, they enter the stage of adaptation. They appear to be, and in fact are, sleek, healthy, strong animals.

Time passes and your rats appear to be doing well. Suddenly, over a short period of time, the rats simply die. They die of chronic stress disease as the various cells in their bodies begin to break down and wear out faster than they can repair themselves and reproduce. Because of the extra hydrocortisone produced during the stress state, they develop stomach ulcers, hemorrhages, and infections, and their adrenal glands give out. This is the same thing that happened to the rats Selye stuck with the needles.

The development of stress disease in humans follows the same three phases, the alarm reaction, adaptation, and exhaustion. There are obvious variations, depending upon the specific stress and the target organ or tissue involved in the stress reaction.

The concept that food or air pollution can cause stress-related disease is at least fifty years old. When I was a freshman in medical school, in 1945, we heard about this crazy professor across town at Northwestern. He was claiming to cure schizophrenics by having them move to the suburbs and live in houses with electric or wood heat. He had the idea that hydrocarbon fumes from automobile exhaust and from coal and gas furnaces caused some people to become schizophrenic. Placed in a clean environment, free from hydrocarbon fumes, he claimed, they became normal. Given a whiff or two of gasoline, they would redevelop their schizophrenic symptoms within a matter of minutes. In other words, their insanity could be turned off and on, like a light.

The professor who told us about this laughed and laughed at the idea. He laughed in spite of the fact that it worked and had been carefully documented in a highly scientific fashion. The "crazy" professor happened to be Dr. Theron Randolph, who was a specialist in both allergy and internal medicine. As I remember the story, he was eventually forced to leave Northwestern because his research and ideas did not conform to what was considered standard, accepted medicine. Randolph moved to southern Illinois and opened his own institute, where he continued to do research and treat patients, free from prejudicial attitudes.

Randolph, Philpott, and those other brave leaders in the field have developed entirely new concepts of the causes, diagnosis, and treatment of many diseases heretofore poorly understood by the medical profession.

The classic method of identifying the environmental stressor causing a particular disease is to admit the patient to an environmentally clean hospital—one with electric heat, no plastics, nobody wearing perfume, etc. The patient is given nothing to eat for five days and only spring water to drink. Usually on the fifth day the symptoms are gone. The patient is then given test meals consisting of single foods and observed closely to see what symptoms recur. He or she is also tested with hydrocarbons, plastics, and other substances commonly found in the environment.

After the testing, a diet and an environment are designed to eliminate and avoid those things to which the patient reacted. Usually, it takes about two or three weeks to work it all out. The patient will remain symptom free and well as long as he or she avoids the offending substance.

A lesson to be learned is that our bodies are not geared to eat the same proteins, carbohydrates, and fats from the same animals and plants, meal after meal, day after day, year after year. Fifty million years ago, our prehistoric ancestors ate what was available. Whatever grasses were in head, they ate the seed. They ate every kind of animal they could kill, from ants and grubs to mastodons. Then came farming and the domestication of animals. This change effectively narrowed the food choices and we began eating what we raised. We have come to the point that we now eat corn and wheat in one form or another at every meal, and beef and milk products at least once or twice daily. We have simply stressed the digestive and metabolic systems of our bodies to death—or at least to disease.

Let us consider an example of how a maladaptive food stress disease evolves. Assume a newborn baby is given a cow's-milk formula and reacts to the protein in the formula with gas, cramps, and diarrhea. This alarm reaction is diagnosed by the doctor as colic. Most likely, the baby will be placed on a soybean formula and everything will be fine. After a while, the mother gives the baby a bit of pudding or cereal with cow's milk, and in this small amount the baby tolerates it. As he continues to receive more milk-containing foods, he begins to adapt by whatever mechanisms his intestine uses to adapt. Eventually, he is drinking regular milk and the doctor announces he has outgrown his colic. In a sense, this is true, but more accurately, the child has now entered the stage of adaptation.

Time passes, perhaps fifteen or twenty years or more. Gradually, the adaptive mechanisms begin to fail, and he starts having some symptoms of gas and cramps. He goes to his doctor, but nothing can be found to explain the symptoms. X-rays and tests are all normal, so the doctor looks for some other explanation. Together, they decide he is working too hard and arrive at the diagnosis of a nervous or spastic colon. The doctor prescribes some pills to relax the muscles of the gut and gives advice about easing off a bit at the office.

Meanwhile, the body is trying to adapt. This is a dynamic process that ebbs and flows, depending upon the amount of stressor consumed and the ability of the body to adjust and adapt. Perhaps he has been picking up some weight, so he cuts back on ice cream for a bedtime snack and he gets better, but he attributes this to the medicine and the relaxation and not to decreasing his intake of milk products. Whatever the circumstances, the disease process tends to wax and wane over a period of months or years. Eventually, the lining of the colon, which has been chronically injured over the years, starts to ulcerate and bleed. He may have as many as fifty or sixty bloody stools a day. Now the doctor is sure of the diagnosis. The ulcers are visible on X-ray and through the colonoscope. He announces to the patient that he has ulcerative colitis. When the patient asks the cause of this potentially fatal disease he is told that the cause is unknown.

The doctor, however, knows what to do. He prescribes a sulfa drug to combat infection in the ulcers of the colon, steroids to reduce inflammation, and, more than likely, supplementary feedings to offset the weight loss due to the diarrhea. The feeding supplements usually take the form of milkshakes, eggnog, or prescription supplements based largely on cow's milk. This is the standard accepted care for ulcerative colitis. In any case, there is little chance the doctor will identify the offending food, milk in this case, and put the patient on a diet devoid of milk and milk products. When the standard accepted treatment fails, and it will, the surgeon is called in to remove his colon and give him a ileostomy, and he is cured. Yeah, you bet he is! How lucky! He won't ever have to worry about being constipated again, or for that matter hemorrhoids, either.

If the offending food, whatever it may be, is eliminated from the diet, the disease simply goes into remission. In other words, the patient gets well. Once the offending food is eliminated, the gas, cramps, and diarrhea usually subside within four or five days. The ulcers will heal, and all the bleeding will stop in another week to ten days. The colitis will remain in remission as long as the patient refrains from eating the offending food. It is just as simple as that. It really is. If he is stupid enough to resume eating the food that is the trigger for the stress reaction, he'll promptly get his ulcerative colitis back.

This whole disease process is so important that I want to cite a number of case histories. Then I'll explain how most of you can test yourself with a minimum of help. I had eleven cases of ulcerative colitis in my practice which I treated in this manner. All but one were due to milk or beef or a combination of the two. The remaining case was due to corn. All of the cases remained in remission. The case in remission the longest was, obviously, the first. She had been well for fifteen years at the time I left practice. The others were diagnosed through the years and observed for lesser periods of time. The last one was caused by corn. She had been well for six months when I retired. Hers is the case I will relate in detail.

Mary's was my last case of colitis, for my colleagues in the clinic had forbidden me to do any more of this kind of work. Consequently, I had to do it on the sly and only with the few patients I could trust to keep the secret and not expose what I was doing. Mary had been diagnosed as having ulcerative colitis by a specialist in gastroenterology a number of years before coming to the clinic where I worked. She was in a chronic stage of the disease but continued to have abdominal pain and one to three bloody stools a day. Because of my experience, with the preceding cases all being caused by beef or milk, I told her it was likely her problem was triggered by these foods. I advised her strongly to avoid them at all costs. I did not test her, for I was not confident she would refrain from making some remark at the hospital where she worked and expose me.

A month passed and she was no better. I really gave her a hard time, for I doubted she was following the diet. She assured me she had not had any beef or milk since I had instructed her to avoid them. Obviously, they were not the cause.

"Well, corn is the most common food to cause reactions," I said. "Let's try stopping corn and corn products."

"Oh, I can't eat corn," she exclaimed. "It goes through me like a dose of salts. I might as well take a laxative."

I pointed out to her that she ate corn products at every meal in the form of corn oil, corn oil margarine, corn syrup, corn fillers, and the like. I cautioned her that she would have to become a label reader, reading the list of ingredients on everything she ate, if she were to eliminate corn completely. She accomplished the task and in one week when she returned to see me, the symptoms, including the bloody stools, were entirely gone. I had her purposely eat corn at one meal as a confirmatory test. Within twenty minutes she developed violent abdominal cramps and had several bloody bowel movements.

Henry was a man who came to me for a physical exam. His history gave no hint of his skin problem. He was found to have high blood pressure and as the examination proceeded I had him remove his underwear. His jockey shorts were glued to his scrotum with dried blood and serum.

"My God, Henry, why didn't you tell me about this?" His scrotum actually resembled a piece of raw, bloody meat. There was nothing that remotely looked like skin. The surface was deeply cracked, oozing blood and serum.

"Oh, I forgot," he replied. "It's been that way for about fifteen years. I've gone to dozens of skin specialists and used about every ointment and medicine there is, but nothing helps."

I tested him and found he reacted to corn. Meanwhile, I referred him to an excellent dermatologist who prescribed a couple of things but to no avail. He returned to see me for a blood pressure check. It was normal with the medicine I had prescribed. Then I sat down with him and talked about the possibility of his skin problem being due to a maladaptive reaction to corn. He agreed to try eliminating all corn and corn products for a month to see what would happen.

Two months passed before he returned. His blood pressure was normal and I asked about his scrotum. He told me he was cured. Seeing is believing, so I had him drop his pants. There was a perfectly normal scrotum. He related that on the fourth or fifth day the itching had stopped. He said he could hardly remember not itching. It took another week for the cracks to stop oozing and begin to seal over. He said it had been just the last ten days or so that the normal pigment in the skin had returned. In order to convince himself, I suggested, he should eat some corn at one meal and see what would happen.

"I've already done that, Doc," he answered. "A couple of weeks ago I ate some corn on the cob. In about ten minutes, I was itching like mad, and in a half hour the skin was all swollen and had begun to split and bleed. I'll never do that again."

Betty was an adult onset diabetic. She was in her late fifties and, even with medicine, her fasting blood sugars were in the 250 range. I worked with her for a couple of years trying to get better control of her diabetes. But we weren't getting anywhere. Finally, she asked if there wasn't something else to try.

"Well, adult onset diabetes is caused by a food reaction. Something you're eating is making you diabetic. If you are really interested, I can test you, find out what food it is. Eliminate the food, and your diabetes might go away."

"You're crazy!" she exclaimed.

"So tell me something we don't already know." We both laughed. "Do you want to try it or do you want to just sit there being an overweight diabetic and call me names?"

She listened to my explanation of stress-related disease and decided she had nothing to lose. She tested positive for both corn and coffee. She announced she could not start the day without her morning coffee. After some good-natured bickering I instructed her concerning the diet and told her to stop her diabetes medicine. She was strictly to avoid coffee and all corn and corn products for one week.

At the end of one week I had her fasting blood sugar tested. It was a nice, normal 108. I had her drink a cup of black coffee and re-tested her blood sugar at the end of one hour. It had risen to 385 and at the end of two hours was still 290. She was impressed. A few days later, we did the same thing using corn. Her fasting sugar was 105. An hour after eating half of a can of corn, it was up to 475 and was still 435 at the end of the second hour.

She argued that corn was a high carbohydrate vegetable and this must account for the extremely high sugars. Declaring she was too stubborn for her own good, I had her return a third time. Again, her fasting blood sugar was normal. This time I had her drink a glass of water into which I had dissolved no less than twelve packets of table sugar. Table sugar comes from sugar cane rather than corn. One hour after drinking the syrup, her blood sugar was only 145, which is a normal rise. At the end of the second hour it was down to 110 as it should have been.

"Good, I'm going out and have a piece of pie."

"Not if it's store bought, or from a restaurant," I cautioned. "Canned fruit is usually sweetened with corn sugar. Go home and make one from scratch using table sugar."

When I left the clinic a year later, she was on no medicine. She was avoiding coffee and corn, and her blood sugars were normal. Betty was no longer a diabetic.

One afternoon, a very pretty young lady came to see me. Her good looks were marred by patches of red scaly skin all over her face and body. It looked like psoriasis, but she had the lesions on her face and portions of her body not usual for the disease. She had come seeking a stronger ointment for her skin problem. As it turned out, she had seen a dermatologist a year before. He had done a skin biopsy, and the pathology report had confirmed the diagnosis of psoriasis. I talked with

her, explaining I knew of nothing better than the cream she was cur-
rently using. Then I approached her about the possibility that her psoriasis was caused by a reaction to some food she was eating on a regular
basis. She was anxious to see what would happen. She tested positive
for only one food—egg. I advised her to quit eating eggs, warning her
to read labels to make certain egg was not an ingredient in prepared
sauces and batters. She assured me no egg would pass her lips.
Explaining that a chronic condition like psoriasis would not clear up
overnight, I gave her an appointment for two weeks hence.

When she walked into my office two weeks later, I could
hardly believe my eyes. There was not a single blemish on her skin,
anywhere. Her complexion was as clear as a newborn baby's.
Subsequently, at my direction, she ate two eggs. She related to me
that within a half hour she was itching slightly and red blotches and
patches had popped up all over her face and body. The next day,
they were gone. Her psoriasis never returned.

In my practice, I had the following cases caused by maladaptive food reactions:

- ELEVEN CASES OF ULCERATIVE COLITIS—*one due to corn, ten
  due to milk or beef or both*
- TWO CASES OF MULTIPLE SCLEROSIS—*both due to wheat*
- ONE CASE OF ECZEMA—*due to corn*
- ONE CASE OF PSORIASIS—*due to egg*
- TWO CASES OF RHEUMATOID ARTHRITIS—*one due to beef, one
  due to tomato and all members of the melon family*
- ONE CASE OF MYASTHENIA GRAVIS—*due to corn*
- TWO CASES OF PARANOID SCHIZOPHRENIA—*one due to tobac-
  co and wheat, one due to tomato and cane sugar*
- ONE CASE OF ENDOGENOUS DEPRESSION—*due to milk*

There could have been more cases, but for two problems. I
had been doing this openly for about three and one-half years when

my colleagues suddenly demanded that I quit or leave the clinic, since my procedures did not conform to standard medical practice. It mattered not that I had this rather impressive group of patients who were essentially cured from these "incurable" diseases. Furthermore, I had begun to get some referrals from doctors outside the clinic. However, I was being different, and my colleagues' rigid belief system was not prepared to accept "different" any longer.

The other problem was the attitude of the patients themselves. Although I had one case of diabetes which was arrested by avoiding corn and coffee, there were fifteen or twenty other diabetics I had approached concerning this concept, and none was remotely interested in trying it out. I would tell them about maladaptive food reactions, saying it might not work but avoiding some food for a week or two couldn't do any harm. It was free, there was no risk of side effects, really nothing to lose. None of the other people was interested in discussing the proposal, much less trying it. Other patients with other diseases I knew to be caused by maladaptive food reactions were just as disinterested in seeing if they could be cured.

This brings us to a major problem in health care. Most patients are unwilling to accept much responsibility for their health. They will consent to a needed operation or take medicine—at least some medicine part of the time—but that's as far as their involvement will go. Every one of you ought to spend some time thinking that statement over. It reminds me of the story about the difference between involvement and commitment: In a breakfast of ham and eggs, the hen was involved, but the pig was committed. Patients need to be committed to good health.

One of the problems many in the medical profession have with the concept of maladaptive food reactions is that they have been called allergies. Skin tests, which are done to determine other allergies such as ragweed sensitivity, are not effective in identifying food reactions. This is the reason that most allergists refuse to accept the fact that food can cause these conditions. These stress diseases, not being true allergies, do not involve the antigen-antibody mechanism that is involved when one has a true allergy, such as a reaction to horse serum or ragweed. It was a mistake to call these stress diseases "allergies" in the first place. The tissue damage in the stress illnesses is caused by certain types of white blood cells breaking apart in the presence of the offending food. The digestive enzymes contained within the white blood cells cause a reaction in the tissues of the shocked organ. The damage somewhat resembles a chronic allergic reaction.

Before the testing, first understand that your body is an electromagnetic field. Anything disturbing the field causes the body to become physically weaker. This weakness can be demonstrated by testing any muscle for its relative strength. Disturb the energy field and the muscle tests weak. Stop the disturbance and the muscle strength immediately returns. So far so good.

Second, there are two places on the body surface which have the ready ability to recognize substances that are "bad" for you. If a "harmful" substance touches either of these areas, your energy field is disturbed and you become weak. These two places are the palm of the hand and the inside of the mouth. The reason for this is unknown, but I have a theory. Surprised?

I believe this phenomenon is the trace of a primitive protective reflex. Most animals gather food or anchor it with their front feet while eating. Since the skin on the bottoms of the front feet has the ability to recognize harmful substances, as the creature begins to eat he will feel weak and wander off to eat something else. With the lining of the mouth possessing the same property, he has a second line of defense. Humans have a small residual of this ancient protective reflex.

Remember, we are talking about an electromagnetic field, so a piece of iron or steel held in the hand will disturb the field and cause weakness. Iron certainly is not bad for you, it simply affects magnetic fields. Therefore, you can use a piece of iron to demonstrate the effect.

You will need someone to help, since you cannot test your own muscle strength. One convenient muscle to use is your deltoid. This is the muscle over your shoulder joint that holds your arm out from your side. Sit or stand with your arm held out sideways at a right angle from your body. Then have your helper push down on your arm while you do your best to resist and keep your arm sticking straight out. Your helper should apply steady, increasing pressure until he or she overcomes your muscle strength, causing your arm to go down. When this happens, both of you should get a good "feel" for just how strong your deltoid muscle is.

Now, place a piece of iron in your opposite hand. Anything made of iron will do—a paper clip, a single staple from a staple machine, or even a pocketknife. While you have the iron object in your hand, do the muscle test again. You and your helper will detect a definite weakness.

(I should say that there is an exception in which the opposite is true—in which holding the iron will make you stronger. This is caused by a reversal of energy flow in the acupuncture meridians and is known as being "switched." If a piece of iron, such as the nosepiece on your glasses or a belt buckle, is crossing your midline, touching the skin, remove it and test again. There are other causes, too, so if you continue to be switched, consult a good chiropractor who is familiar with kinesiology.)

Normally, while you have the iron in your hand, your helper won't have to push down as hard to overcome your strength. You will feel an obvious decrease in your ability to resist. Magic, huh? No way. Fact! The same thing happens when you hold medicine or a bit of food to which you are sensitive or allergic.

When you test food, test one food at a time. If you wish to test beef do not use beef hash for, depending upon the cook, you will be testing potato, onion, pepper, and whatever else the cook put in the hash. Bread contains milk, yeast, and shortening, as well as wheat. Flour is appropriate for testing wheat. Use your head and think.

A small number of food items are responsible for perhaps ninety percent of all food reactions. The reason is that we eat them in one form or another several times a week or even more often. They are, in no particular order:

Corn	*Onion*
Wheat	*Yeast*
Milk	*Coffee*
Beef	*Pepper*
Egg	*Chocolate*
Potato	*Tomato*

Tobacco is often a cause of stress diseases. Those of you who do not smoke should also test with tobacco because you inhale it so frequently from those who do. Test these and all other foods that you eat at least three or four times a week. It's wise to test everything. Likely, you will discover the food you like best will be the one to which you are sensitive, because an addictive element is also at work in the development of food-related illness.

After you have determined the foods that cause you to become weak, simply exclude those items from your diet for a period of at least one week. By exclusion, I mean total, absolute exclusion, not even a drop or a crumb. Corn, wheat, milk, and egg are in nearly everything, so you need to become a label reader. Corn sugar is so labeled, so if the label says "sugar" it means cane sugar, which is ordinary table sugar. Non-dairy creamers are mostly corn syrup solids. Most canned soup contains wheat flour to thicken the broth to make it appear richer. It can be very tricky, but you don't have to be a doctor to do it.

Keep in mind that you may have unnoticed symptoms that are not part of the condition you're trying to cure. If you have rheumatoid arthritis and test positive to both beef and milk, the milk may be responsible for your post-nasal drip while the beef is triggering the arthritis.

After being free of the suspected food(s) for a period of four or five days, your body will have cleared itself. This is the reason that dialysis of the blood is effective in relieving symptoms for short periods of time. Occasionally, reactions to wheat may take up to two weeks to clear. If the food you eliminated is the one responsible for your troubles, your symptoms should be gone. Even chronic diseases such as arthritis should show a marked decrease in the intensity or even the absence of the symptoms within seven days.

Now comes the acid test. Choose a day on which you can afford to have a flare-up of your illness. For breakfast, eat nothing but the one suspected food. Don't eat anything else. Then sit back and wait to see what happens. It's probably a good idea to have a pencil and paper to jot down everything that occurs—from an itch to a headache, nausea, a runny nose, everything. It won't take long; often, symptoms will start within a few minutes. Sometimes, it may require an hour or two.

During the time your body was free of exposure to the offending food, it reverted to the alarm stage of the disease. Therefore, the recurring symptoms are often more violent and severe than the chronic problem you have been experiencing. Don't worry, for they will subside within a few hours. Should you have no reaction, eat a second meal of the same food at noon. This is especially true of wheat reactions. Wheat sometimes requires several challenges to trigger a response. If you had no reaction with the first food, or after the reaction has fully subsided, you can test the second item, assuming you reacted to more than one thing.

There are more considerations. Sometimes, whole food groups are involved; because the plants and animals within the group are so closely related, the proteins, starches, and fats have a similar chemical makeup. People who react to beef very often are unable to eat lamb, deer, buffalo, or elk. All are members of the antelope family. One of my patients developed a classic rheumatoid arthritis after eating lots of watermelon in an attempt to lose some weight. It turned out she reacted to cucumbers and all the melons in the entire cucumber family.

Personally, I have a whole group of symptoms caused by beef. All my life I had been troubled with a lot of intestinal gas which completely disappeared after eliminating beef from my diet. After being on a beef-free diet for about six weeks, I decided it was high time I tested myself. It was Christmas and my wife and I had gone out for dinner. The restaurant was serving a beautiful standing rib roast, so I ordered it. It was delicious.

By the time I was finishing the meal I had been forced to loosen my belt and had begun to have abdominal cramps. We hurried home, which was a short, ten-minute drive. Somewhere along the way, I had to unzip my pants. I got home and ran to the house holding my trousers, heading for the john. My wife looked at me, saying, "My God, you look like you're nine months pregnant!" I spent the next three hours having an explosive, bloody diarrhea.

Along with the hemorrhagic colitis, I developed a strange headache with an anxiety attack. I had experienced this particular headache all my life but thought it to be a tension headache. I'd slept with my head on a heating pad half my life. I hadn't missed the headache during the six weeks I had been off beef. As soon as it recurred I recognized it as being associated with my beef reaction. In addition, my chronic constipation exists no longer. I wish I had all the money I spent on bran trying in vain for a bit of help and even one soft stool. Needless to say, I no longer eat beef.

Some of you are thinking that with your arthritis or multiple sclerosis, your shoulders are too weak or painful to hold your arm out to the side, much less have someone pushing on it. What will you do? There is a simple answer. Have your spouse or a friend do the test for you, using his or her arm instead. You see, a disturbance in one person's energy field will affect another's energy field if they are holding hands. A third person is needed to do the test. You hold the food in one hand and hold hands with the first helper. The third person tests the strength of the helper with whom you are holding hands. Your field disturbance will be transferred to the person touching your palm, who will test weak if you react to the test food. The same method can be used to check infants or children when they are unable or unwilling to cooperate.

Give it a try. After all, what do you have to lose? If it works and you feel better, then great. Avoid the food and enjoy better health. If it doesn't help for some reason, at the worst you are right back where you started. The only cases I have personally observed that were unsuccessful were individuals who, I suspect, did not follow the diet.

One woman of my acquaintance started developing a typical rheumatoid arthritis. Her hands were most affected, which is commonly true with this kind of arthritis. Her knuckle joints and the second joints of the fingers were markedly swollen, tender, and red. She was having pain in her elbows and knees as well and had experienced symptoms for several months when she came to me. The only food she tested positive for was beef, so I suggested she quit eating beef for a couple of weeks and see if it helped. Within a week, the redness, swelling, and pain were completely gone from all her joints. We agreed it had been a dramatic response, and I urged her to continue avoiding beef in all forms.

A few days later, she approached me in a rather hostile manner, asking if she had to refrain from eating beef the rest of her life? I told her that after about six months she might be able to eat beef once in a while, providing it was no more frequent than once a week. She was obviously very unhappy, in spite of her joints' being normal.

About two weeks later, I heard that her arthritis had flared up again. I inquired if she had resumed eating beef, and she assured me that she had not. Meanwhile, unbeknown to me, she had consulted an arthritis specialist who prescribed some medicine for her. Sometime later, I ran into her and again had an opportunity to inquire as to how she was doing. She did not mention the trip to the rheumatologist nor the medicine she was taking. She informed me, angrily, that her arthritis had recurred in spite of her continuing to avoid beef. I glanced at her hands. She was right about the flare up. Her knuckles and finger joints were very swollen and red, worse than before, and she was having a lot of difficulty using her hands in her work. Later, a mutual acquaintance told me that on several occasions she had seen the woman eating a hamburger while telling several people with whom she was having lunch that I was a crackpot and didn't know what I was talking about.

Some people would rather be ill. Perhaps she valued the sympathy her arthritis brought her more than the benefits of being pain and arthritis free. A little illness can be a marvelous thing, providing it doesn't prevent you from doing what you want. It can also be used as an excuse to avoid unwanted tasks. Think about all the people who are admired for their ability to accomplish some task while "fighting" some dreaded and painful disease. Wow! It doesn't get any better than that. There is no illness so terrible that the person does not receive certain benefits from it.

A word of caution about the advice in this chapter: Do not expect to recover fully from all your disability. The "cure" simply stops the disease from progressing and puts it into a stage of inactivity. If your joints are all crippled and deformed by arthritis they are not going to straighten out completely and become normal again. That's not realistic. Some of the swelling will subside, and the pain should largely go away. With the decrease in pain, the function should also improve to some extent. What more could you expect? Experiment, give it a try, have fun, enjoy life, and above all don't be afraid. As Oscar Wilde said, "Life is too important to be taken seriously."

PSYCHOSOMATIC
DISEASES

ASK MOST DOCTORS what a psychosomatic disease is, and more than likely you will get an answer along these lines: It is a disease caused by the imagination—real but not real—sort of in the mind. Actually, most, if not all, diseases are psychosomatic in origin. These illnesses fall under three groupings, although there is considerable overlapping. Two of the groups can be defined according to the emotional environment in which they develop. The third group encompasses the other two and, in fact, just about everything else that goes wrong with people. To understand the first two, it is necessary to consider the various ways we relate to life situations.

Most people have no clear understanding of why they are here or what purpose their existence serves. Often, people think of life's trials as burdens heaped upon them by God, paying them back for their sins. In truth, the problems of life are glorious opportunities we set up for ourselves to experience growth of character. They are each a chance to learn and attain wisdom. Unfortunately, the vast majority of people handle these life stresses rather inappropriately, to say the very least.

Any change is stress. We tend to think of stress as a bad event, such as wrecking the car, flunking a test, or the death of a loved one. These are, indeed, stressful, but so are falling in love, winning the lottery, and being promoted at your job. Whatever the stress, it calls upon the whole being to adjust, and many of us don't do that very well. I have a Willie Nelson tape on which he sings "I've survived every situation, knowing when to freeze and when to run—." That pretty well sums up the options in life. We can withdraw into ourselves and freeze, so to speak, or we can do something, such as run or attack. Put into the context of motion, to move or not to move are the two basic choices. Even the simplest forms of life have these options. Expressed in terms of emotional response, these options are identical with anxiety and depression.

Observe someone who is anxious or frightened and you will see him fidget, drum his fingers on the table, or pace the floor. Anxious people just can't sit still. When really frightened, they will run away if they can or, if escape is impossible, they are apt to attack.

On the other hand, a person who is depressed withdraws. She doesn't want to be involved with her environment, or with anything else. If given a choice she would prefer to crawl into a corner or into bed, curl up, and become immobile.

Now, there are times when being anxious or depressed is appropriate. If you are being threatened by your boss and about to lose your job, or if a mugger has a knife to your throat, fear and anxiety are certainly logical and appropriate emotions to exhibit. If your spouse just died, you have the right to be depressed until you have had a chance to grieve and make some adjustments. Where humankind gets into trouble is by borrowing trouble, wonder, and worry. Humans have the capability of maintaining themselves in a constant state of anxiety or depression. And this continuous, chronic, abnormal emotional state sets the framework for a multitude of medical conditions.

Imagine a deer feeding in a forest meadow. He hears a noise and immediately tenses. A lot of automatic responses take place in his body. His heart quickens, his muscles tense for a fast getaway, digestion stops, blood vessels constrict, and many other things occur, all geared to escaping or being attacked. The deer waits—no more strange noises, so he puts the situation out of his mind, and his body goes back to normal. He could not survive in a continual state of fear. Prey animals do not live in constant fear of the predator. I've been in East Africa. Wildebeest do not tremble with terror when they see a lion. Mostly, they appear to ignore each other. Being alert to danger does not imply fearing danger. If the deer were like most of us, he would be wondering and worrying about all the terrible possibilities of what might have been. Was that noise a cougar or a man with a gun? What if it's sneaking up at this very moment? Maybe the hunter already has him in his sights! What if he's killed or wounded? What if? What if? What if? You all know the process. You go through it every day of your life.

We have already agreed that anxiety and depression are normal responses at times. What gets us into trouble is the sustained emotion. At some point, the system says, "That's enough!" or "This has gone on long enough," and ends the process. Within each person's physiologic makeup is an end point or benchmark, which establishes a limit to how long these emotions should continue and the depth of the emotional response. If we exceed these limits, we start to pay a price in terms of the acute and chronic physical changes we call illness.

Physiologists tell us that thoughts and emotions are transmitted to the body through the "primitive" portion of the brain common to all animals. This area is made up of the midbrain, thalamus, and hypothalamus. It is this portion of the brain in which the so-called basic emotions, such as fear, anger, and hunger, are transmitted to the body to produce appropriate physiologic changes. This area of the brain connects physically to the rest of the body via nerve pathways in the spinal cord and the autonomic nervous system, and through the hormones of the pituitary gland.

The autonomic nervous system has two parts. One tends to stimulate those cells to which it is attached, and the other part sedates or calms the activity of those cells. Acting together, both parts serve as a sort of governing mechanism, keeping many body systems functioning in a dynamic balance. For example, one set of nerves causes arteries to constrict, while the other causes them to dilate. One set causes your mouth to water; the other set causes the saliva to cease flowing and your mouth becomes dry.

The pituitary gland is an organ located at the base of the brain. The back part is connected to the brain by nerves and the front part is unconnected, receiving information by chemicals produced in the hypothalamus. The front portion, or anterior pituitary, secretes hormones that stimulate other endocrine glands in the body to secrete their hormones. A hormone is a chemical that produces effects on certain cells within the body. Perhaps the best way to explain it is to give an example.

A hormone called thyroid stimulating hormone (TSH) is produced by the pituitary gland. TSH travels though the blood and reaches the thyroid gland located in your neck, just beneath your voice box. TSH attaches to the surface of the thyroid cells and causes them to release their hormone, called thyroxin, into the bloodstream. Thyroxin then goes, via the bloodstream, to every cell in the body, increasing its rate of metabolism or activity. As the thyroxin level rises, it causes the pituitary gland to shut down its production of TSH. In this way, a constant balance is maintained between the levels of TSH and thyroxin and the metabolic "needs" of the body's cells at any given moment. This is a somewhat simplified account, but it illustrates the point I wish to make.

The pituitary gland makes a number of different hormones, but the ones we are most concerned about for the purpose of this discussion are growth hormone, called somatotropic hormone (STH), and adrenocorticotropic hormone (ACTH). Growth hormone acts upon every cell in the body to stimulate activity directed toward growth and maintenance of the cells. This is called an anabolic effect. It stimulates the immune system to fend off attacks by bacteria and viruses, to destroy foreign proteins, etc. ACTH, on the other hand, acts on the cortical cells of the adrenal gland to cause the secretion of hydrocortisone and other hormones, namely sex hormones. Hydrocortisone does a number of things that help defend the individual during short-term stress. In doing this task, some of the effects actually interfere with the body's ability to fight infections and heal wounds. Other effects of hydrocortisone are an increase of acid production in the stomach, the breakdown of intracellular proteins, which are converted to glucose, the suppressed formation of scar tissue, and many others.

Now, let's take an example and think through to effects that might occur in a person who is always frightened and worried, anticipating grave consequences from every little thing that comes along. This reaction of chronic anxiety causes an increased production of ACTH with an effect on the body as though the person were taking tablets of hydrocortisone every day.

Let's think about this physiologic function. There is certainly a chronic over-production of ACTH, which causes the adrenal cortex to produce more hydrocortisone than it ordinarily would. A couple of other things happen as well. First, the target cells that are affected by the hydrocortisone become more sensitive to the effects of the hydrocortisone. As a result, even normal levels of hormone produce a far more dramatic response than would usually occur. Second, and even more important, *all the cells in the body are independently aware of the emotional attitude of the person and respond on their own.* Thus, if we are suddenly placed in a dangerous situation—such as nearly being struck by a car or a near miss from a shotgun blast—every cell in the body is instantly aware of the danger and acts accordingly in its specific manner. A few moments later, the body physiology, directed by the nervous system and the hormones, catches up with the situation, supporting the cells of the body in their response to the attack.

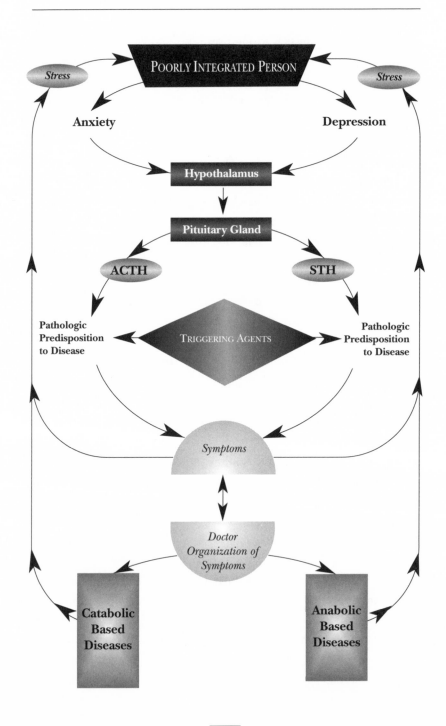

Back to our hypothetical case. At this point, the person is not physically sick. He is, however, primed and ready. I call this phase the state of being pathologically predisposed to an illness, but not just any illness. He is predisposed to specific illnesses as determined by the long-term effects of the hydrocortisone, the particular triggering agent that happens along, and the reaction and attitude of the physician.

Symptoms are usually the result of an interaction between the body of the patient and some triggering agent. These agents take the form of bacteria, viruses, foods, chemicals, toxins, and many other things widely considered by the medical profession to be the "causes" of disease. Doctors have been obsessed from the beginning with finding the specific *cause* of disease and have confused the triggering agents with the *true* causes.

If you contract a respiratory infection and the doctor's diagnosis is pneumonia, you probably did not catch it from someone with pneumonia. If you gather a lot of people off the street, line them up, and culture their throats, lots of disease organisms, including pneumonia germs, will be found in most of the cultures. The fault, if you want to think of it in those terms, and the reason you got pneumonia lie within your body defense mechanisms *and your expectations.* Something went haywire, allowing the bacteria that are *always* present to get a foothold and start multiplying to produce the infection. I do not discount the possibility of your becoming ill as a result of being exposed to an overwhelming infection from someone else. But I do propose that this really doesn't happen very often. Epidemics do occur, but that is a different story.

There is a fascinating interaction between the doctor and the patient which is essential to the development of a disease. In 1957, a remarkable book was published entitled *The Doctor, His Patient and the Illness.* It was written by an English physician named Michael Balint. I owe the basic concepts of the following revelations to him, although I have modified and added to them based upon my experience. Balint says that the patient, not being able to cope with life stresses or to react in a truly mature fashion, converts his problem to a symptom and then takes the symptom to the doctor for approval.

So our person who is constantly anxious develops a symptom. In our hypothetical example, let us assume it is indigestion resulting from excessive stomach acid caused by the hydrocortisone. He then takes his indigestion, as though it were an offering, to the doctor for approval. As a result, his doctor becomes an active participant in the formation and organization of the disease.

The doctor is actually a major factor in deciding what illness if any will be developed. The patient may have the symptom, but it is the doctor who will either accept or reject it. She has the power to add importance and validity to the offered symptom. It is her manner, her tone of voice and facial expression, her body language and actions through which the patient receives subtle hints as to whether the doctor is impressed or unconcerned. If the doctor decides to order tests or X-ray studies, she further increases the importance of the symptom. If tests are not obtained, this is a signal that the symptom may not be serious. What's more, if the physician openly rejects the offering, saying something to the effect that the symptom is unimportant, and fails to give the patient a prescription, the patient has several options of response. If the patient is determined that his basic emotional problem must be placated and is equally certain that to be ill is the most appropriate way to deal with the trouble, he must do something else. First, he can produce another symptom, and another, and another, offering them to the doctor until she is satisfied. The doctor's satisfaction is based upon recognition and belief that the symptoms fall into a group she was trained to recognize and is able to name.

The other option for the patient is to take the original symptom from doctor to doctor looking for a physician who will accept the offering as valid, give it the name of a real disease, and start treatment. It is the poor soul who just can't seem to come up with the right combination of symptoms who is known as a hypochondriac, the person whom doctors regard as a "neurotic." There are other people who are not satisfied with one disease. They may have a tremendously stressful life situation and after organizing one illness find it inadequate. They must organize another and another, never coming to grips with the true reality of the situation.

My Uncle Porter graduated from medical school a few years prior to World War I. Once, I heard him relate an incident that had taken place when he was in medical school. A professor introduced a woman for the class to question, obtain a medical history, and arrive at a diagnosis. She was a pathetic individual with dozens of physical ailments and symptoms. She kept saying, over and over, that none of the doctors believed her. Here she was, suffering terribly, and none of the physicians took her symptoms seriously. The professor excused the lady and then went about the class listing all the possible diagnoses the students felt appropriate.

Finally, they asked the teacher what was wrong with her. He replied there was nothing wrong. She wasn't really sick. He reasoned that if the patient had a real disease it would never occur to her that the doctors would not believe her.

To a degree, this is true. Remember when you used to fib to your mother saying, "Why don't you believe me?" The truth is, this particular woman had not yet achieved success in developing the right combination of symptoms or in finding a physician who would accept her symptoms and help *organize* her illness.

Sometimes, the symptoms are such that the patient has already organized his illness without the assistance of a doctor. On other occasions, friends or relatives may assist in its organization, validating the symptoms and naming the disease.

Names are very important. To have true value and be an adequate substitute for the real problem—the incapacity to cope with stress without sustained anxiety or depression—the disease *must* have a defined name.

The treatment prescribed is also of great psychological importance. It is most effective if it—consciously or subconsciously—

conforms to what the patient feels is appropriate. Patients are often quite knowledgeable about what to expect in the way of treatment. They have definite ideas about what is and is not proper. They aren't always right, but, like everyone else, they have opinions. Many patients, for example, are convinced they need an antibiotic to recover from a cold. Colds are virus infections, and antibiotics have no effect upon viruses. The doctor can explain this to the patient, as I have done on countless occasions, but most people will still insist upon receiving an expensive antibiotic and will settle for absolutely nothing less.

Now, this whole process started with the patient's inability to cope with stress in a healthy manner. (Please refer to the diagram on page 62). As each step in the development and organization of the illness unfolds, it acts to *increase* stress. The symptoms are a cause for worry, and after the disease is organized *it* is a further source of concern. Stress builds upon stress in a truly cybernetic system.

Inappropriate, chronic anxiety triggers a catabolic state, inviting illnesses such as infections, peptic ulcers, and cancer. These and others are characterized by the blunting of the body defenses that ward off infections. Thus, the person who is deathly afraid of getting cancer is actually setting himself up for it. Our bodies neutralize and defend against cancer in much the same fashion that they fight infections. The point I am making is that one's attitude toward life does affect one's health and can promote disease. I hope to make this clearer later in this chapter, when I talk of the third mechanism of psychosomatic illness.

Chronic depression, on the other hand, sets us up for a host of different diseases. In the case of depression, the pituitary gland over-produces the hormone that is responsible for stimulating growth when we are young. If the body is deficient in growth hormone, we fail to grow and are known as pituitary dwarfs. After we attain our full growth, the hormone continues to be the most powerful anabolic agent at work in the body. An anabolic agent, among other tasks, stimulates the rebuilding of protein structures inside the cells and storage of food within the cells. The mechanism for the production of depression-supported disease is the same as for anxiety-produced diseases. The person reacts to stress with depression, and excess STH is produced, setting up a pathological predisposition for the illness. Activated by a triggering agent, symptoms develop which are taken to the doctor for approval and the disease is organized by the patient with the help and approval of the doctor.

Let me give you some case histories to illustrate the phenomenon. Balint tells of one family with a number of children who were always ill with strep throats. He said there was not a week without one or more of the kids' coming down sick. The other children in the community had occasional strep infections, too, but with this particular family the children were always ill. Balint and his colleagues looked into the family situation and found that the mother and father were constantly fighting and arguing. In other words, the family was dysfunctional and the kids were in an insecure environment. The children were just plain scared. The doctors started working with the parents, doing some counseling and helping them cope with their problems in a better fashion. As the parents settled down, quit fighting, and started to deal with life stresses in a more mature manner, the children stopped getting sick. They weren't anxious and afraid any longer, their ACTH levels dropped, their immune systems were no longer suppressed, and, as if by magic, no more strep infections.

In my practice, I observed that it was the poor who were usually sick all the time. There were probably a number of factors at work. Usually, their nutrition was not good. This was not due to the amount of money available for food but resulted mostly from poor buying practices and eating habits. It always amazed me to see what these folks used their money and food stamps to buy. Their carts were loaded down with cookies, pop, fancy pickles, candy, sugar-coated cereal whatevers, expensive prepared junk food, TV dinners, bologna, cigarettes, and beer. Obviously, they had enough money to have eaten well if only they'd had the knowledge, planning skills, and discipline to do so.

Usually, the emotional "diet" in the home was as bad as the food. In the days I made house calls, I would observe constant screaming and fighting between the children and the adults in the house. Beds were unmade, the sink was full of dirty pots and dishes, and usually the kids were dirty. What I am describing is not a home where anyone could feel secure. Anxiety was everywhere. I could imagine their adrenal glands pumping out enough hydrocortisone to suppress everyone's immune system within a three-block radius. When I had a family that was relatively affluent in which the members were often sick, it was almost always a dysfunctional family, too.

This effect of hydrocortisone suppressing the immune system can be demonstrated in animals as well. Animals can be rendered more susceptible to infections by giving them small doses of ACTH, or hydrocortisone. The opposite result can be obtained with small amounts of growth hormone. Growth hormone makes the immune system more effective. Years ago, I read an article in which researchers took a bunch of white rats and, through trial and error, determined the number of disease germs injected into the abdominal cavity it took to kill half of them. (This is called the LD50—the lethal dose to fifty percent of the animals.) Half would die, and half would survive. The researchers then pretreated two other groups of rats: one with ACTH and the other with STH. The rats given the ACTH had almost no resistance to the bacteria, dying with an overwhelming infection upon being injected with only a few germs. Only a very few members of the group given the growth hormone were killed by the disease germs. Their immune systems were so pumped up that even huge doses, far beyond the LD50, failed to make them sick. This is exciting stuff!

A fascinating case of my own involved a young lady who had contracted tuberculosis. She was in a TB sanitarium and was doing poorly. The medicine, rest, and good food were not working. She had a large open cavity in her left lung and was quite contagious. Obviously, she could not go home and she was scared to death that she was going to die. With all the ACTH she was producing as a result of that fear, her immune system was depressed and the scar tissue which would ordinarily wall off the cavity was unable to form. A couple of years passed and then, over a period of a few weeks, her mood dramatically changed. She became very depressed. She gave up, stayed in her room, convinced she would never get out of the hospital, much less go home. Her body quit over-producing ACTH and started making a lot of growth hormone as a result of the depression. Her immune system perked up and her fibroblasts started laying down scar tissue, walling off the cavity. Within a month, the cavity was closed, she was no longer contagious, and she was discharged.

Unfortunately, I saw her several months later in my office with a full-blown rheumatoid arthritis. Rheumatoid arthritis is one of the diseases which occurs in individuals who have a pathologic predisposition to disease caused by over-production of growth hormone. This case was particularly interesting because it graphically demonstrated the patient's switching diseases as the emotional response to stress changed from anxiety to depression.

The last, but probably most important and far-reaching, aspect in the development of psychosomatic disease is the effect of the belief system of the patient upon his or her health. Directly or indirectly, through its effect upon the cellular consciousness, belief and expectation cause every human illness and accident. To appreciate the dynamics of the process, it is necessary to understand that the body, mind, and spirit are fused into one dynamic whole. Without becoming too lost in the metaphysical, let me simply state again that *your thoughts and ideas dictate how the cells of your body behave.* If you believe your body is weak and has little resistance, you are apt to catch everything that comes along. This belief will affect the cells in your immune system and every cell of your body, thus making you more susceptible to infections.

This metaphysical effect operates independently of the nerve and hormonal mechanisms we have been discussing. In other words, being depressed or anxious has nothing to do with this mechanism, unless the depression or anxiety is directed toward illness or the possibility of becoming ill. If you believe you are destined to develop heart disease at an early age because your father did, the cells of your arteries and heart will cooperate fully with your subconscious directions. In other words, your bio-consciousness will direct your body physiology to *produce* a heart attack. Some people go through life actually looking for an illness. I have had patients who literally awakened every morning and examined their bodies from head to toe feeling for the most minute lump. The smallest irregularity would bring them running in a panic for me to examine the bump and assure them they were not dying of cancer. People like this are literally programming themselves for illness.

One of the things that struck me most often when I was practicing was the apparent inability of many of my patients to be presented with a problem and not worry about it. I finally decided they had not learned or developed any thought process other than worry. I used to draw a diagram for them, showing the steps needed to solve a problem.

From looking at the various steps, it is apparent there are several places where people get hung up. In his book *Potential*, Hugh Downs talks about the importance of not limiting the options when one is considering a plan of action, no matter how bizarre they may first seem. This is particularly important when you're searching for a solution to a problem. It is just as important to write the list of options down on a piece of paper. The mind often forgets the most viable and creative options in favor of others that seem more standard and acceptable. The second place of difficulty comes when one has determined the best approach to the problem but is unable to take the plunge and act. The final hang-up is the failure to reevaluate the situation to determine whether it has indeed been solved.

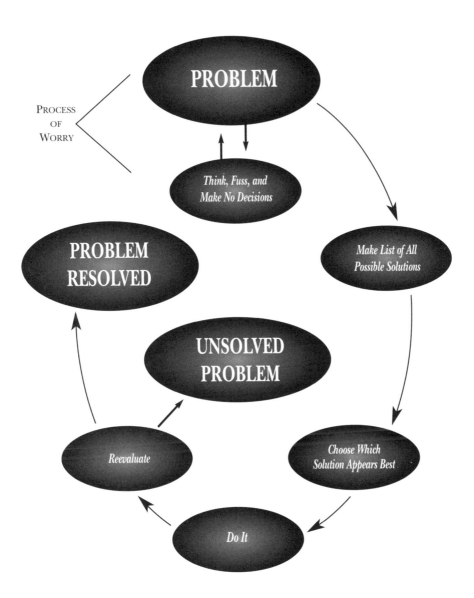

FLOW CHART OF PROBLEM SOLVING

Too often, the planned action is not adequate to the task, yet the individual continues working on a solution that will be only half successful. Nothing should be chiseled in stone.

Oriental philosophy offers much that Western thought does not even pretend to address. There are three basic exercises practiced by Zen followers which can help an individual deal with stress. They are immobility, breath control, and centering. The Zen master will tell you that your body and spirit are one. It is impossible to calm your spirit directly if you are upset. But you can, with practice, control your body. And, by the simple act of quieting your body, your spirit will also be calmed. Try it. If you are upset, try sitting perfectly still. You either have to calm down or fidget. If you will yourself to sit absolutely still, your spirit must become calm as well.

The second exercise is breath control. When we are excited, we breathe faster. If you can make your breath come more slowly and rhythmically, you will find yourself calming down. Learning to control one's breathing is a key to spiritual calm.

The third exercise is called "centering." It is the Zen followers' belief that the center of the soul is in the belly, about two inches below the navel. The Japanese speak of this spot as the center of your being, your *hara*. *Hara* means belly. For this reason, the ritual suicide, *hara-kiri* or *seppuku*, involves cutting the belly. The concept of center has even gotten into Western language. We speak of a well-centered person, or a self-centered or eccentric person. Simply because being centered is so important, I used to urge my most anxious patients to practice an exercise of centering for about ten minutes a day.

To do this, one sits in a chair and thinks of oneself at the center of an imaginary circle. The thing that occupies the center is the essence of the self, that part of our being that is indestructible. To use a hypothetical example, the John of the John Doe would be at the center. John would then push out to the periphery of the circle all the things with which he is involved. He would place the Mr. Doe, his wife, children, relatives, in-laws, friends, home, possessions, job, associations, his bank account, his health, and anything else with which he is attached as far from his self as possible. He would think about all these things until he came to realize that they are not him. They are separate from John. John is not to be identified in terms of John's job, for an example, nor in terms of what he owns. John's ego must release these things as being part of John.

The purpose of the exercise is for John to gain release from his ego's attachment to the activities and associations with which he is involved. The acid test to determine if this detachment has been achieved would be for someone to come to John and say, "Your wife and children have been killed when your car crashed into your house and burned it to the ground. Your relatives, friends and in-laws have abandoned you. You have been fired from your job, and your bank account has been stolen, leaving you penniless. Your bowling team has kicked you out of the league, and the doctor just called saying that you have a fatal disease with only a month to live." To all this, John could reply, "So far, nothing has happened to me." John is still intact. His soul is untouched.

Once John achieves this position, he is free to become even more involved with life. His ego is no longer on the line. If his kid makes the honor roll, John can be happy *for* the child and not because it makes him look better as a parent. If his kid screws up, John is free to give help and advice and not cry, "How can you shame me so?" John thus becomes a better husband, father, and employee, and his bowling score will probably improve now that John doesn't have to prove his worth with every frame he bowls. To the outsider, John will probably seem no different. John will be just as active and busy as before. John will, however, *feel* quite different—free, less has-sled and more wholly in control.

Our bodies break down and grow old for a number of rea-sons. One of these reasons, and not the least important, is that we *expect* them to break down and grow old. Let me give you an exam-ple. Depak Chopra tells of an experiment carried out by a professor at Harvard in about 1985. The professor took a group of one hundred people, all in their seventies and eighties, to a place outside Boston. He divided them into two groups of fifty, making sure they were as nearly identical as possible in age, sex, physical health, etc. The two groups were separated. He instructed the first group to spend the next few days recalling and thinking about their lives, and the events of twenty-five years ago. The second group was told they were to pretend it was 1960. They were to talk of 1960 as if it were the present. When they turned on the radio or TV, they got a taped program from 1960. The newspaper and magazines were from 1960, and they were encouraged to discuss these events as if they were current.

After a few days, an independent observer who had no idea what had been going on was asked to look at the two groups and see if he noticed any differences between them. He reported that he didn't see any difference except that one group was considerably younger than the other. The "younger" group was the one pretending to live in 1960.

So the professor called in the medical laboratory people and started running tests. The tests were those designed to determine physiological age. For instance, the vital capacity of the lungs reaches its peak in adult life. Then, as one grows older, the lungs become stiffer and the vital capacity starts declining at a predictable rate. There are charts which indicate that if one has lost, say, fifteen percent of vital capacity, then the person is a particular age. All in all, they ran about one hundred tests of this type, and every one of the fifty people who had been pretending it was 1960 checked out physiologically to be twenty years younger than they actually were, on every single test!

George Burns said the reason he didn't get old was that he never practiced being old. He claimed that upon reaching sixty, most people start walking old and talking old and thinking old, so that by the time they reached seventy, they have it perfected.

This is not a myth, nor is it some theoretical possibility. It is reality. The people in Chopra's experiment altered their body functions within a few short days. It is apparent that our cells actually function according to our expectations—according, that is, to the specific directions we give them. Earlier in the book, I spoke of epidemics and implied that if people got sick in an epidemic, they were not responsible. Truth is, even in an epidemic with everyone falling ill around us, we have control over whether we become ill. Not everyone gets sick in an epidemic. If you assume that becoming sick is inevitable, then you program your immune system to be less active than it ordinarily would be, and your bio-consciousness gears itself to deliver sickness instead of health. You visualize yourself in bed, perhaps dying of the disease and, in doing so, program yourself for illness and death. Think about it, with most people, the first time they sneeze they mentally throw up their hands in surrender to the cold they assume they are getting, and their body happily cooperates with the virus to provide the symptoms and the disease.

On the other hand, if you do not fall into the trap of expecting to get old or sick, if you continue to be active and interested, continuing to participate fully in life, planning for the future, giving your cellular consciousness directions to structure itself in patterns of youth and vigor, then age and illness can largely be avoided or postponed. If you think of yourself as being vigorously healthy and take care of yourself, avoiding destructive habits and maintaining good nutrition, and if you trust your bio-consciousness, it will comply and you will, more than likely, remain healthy and vigorous.

There are a lot of reasons folks become ill. Some people seek illness, because being sick is a great way to get attention and sympathy and to avoid doing what you don't care to do. A more frequent reason is that people do not realize they have the option of not being sick. They fail to recognize they have the power to refuse to become ill and "just say no"—although it is a bit more complicated than that. They fail to understand that they are literally in the constant process of constructing their bodies and have the power to make them healthy or otherwise. No person becomes ill who does not at some level of their being wish to be so. No person dies who does not wish to die. Nobody is killed in a plane crash or an earthquake, is murdered or shot by a sniper, who does not wish to die. Psychic intent is the determining factor between health and disease, or life and death.

The men of the Tarahumara Indians in central Mexico are famous for their long-distance running. For centuries the various villages have kept in communication by means of runners who run between them carrying news back and forth. It is not unusual for a runner to run forty or fifty miles a day over mountain paths. The interesting thing is that the best runners are not the twenty-year-olds or even those in their thirties. The forty-year-old men can outrun them any day. The fifty-year-old runners are even better, and the best of all are in their sixties. Even then they do not peak, but maintain their stamina for years.

Physiologists have studied these runners, looking for the secret to their continued ability to run these distances even when they are old men. After all the tests were done, it boiled down to one thing: It is the clear belief among the Tarahumara Indians that the older a man gets, the better he is at running. Their bodies and their abilities simply follow their belief system.

You represent yourself in time and space as a fusion of a spirit and a conscious mind with a physical body. Anything that affects any one of these three manifestations necessarily affects your whole being. It is obvious that all three aspects of your being must participate in the healing process, but the process of healing is far more than consenting to an operation, taking some medicine, or even wishing you were well. It requires more than passively accepting the assistance of an outsider. It involves a spiritual and cellular agreement to the total process of healing. True, a person is a spirit with a conscious mind and a body and all need to be addressed in the heal-

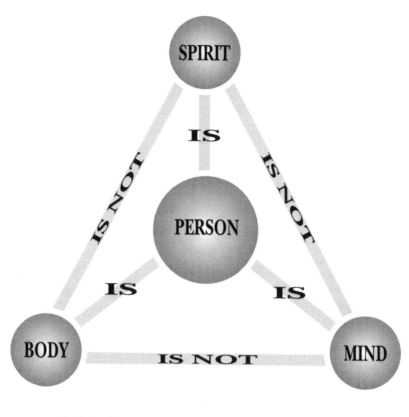

DIAGRAM OF A PERSON

ing adventure. But, in addition, the part that is usually omitted is that the cells themselves need to be involved at their own level of consciousness. To understand the mechanism, a look at a deeper metaphysical level of being is paramount.

All illnesses and injuries are, at every level of your being, psychosomatic in origin. The physical body is a construction of your consciousness. You construct it with your thoughts from inside outward. Your body is not a living thing that your soul hopped into and which somehow runs along on its own according to instructions from the genes. Your beliefs and thoughts literally form the energy field that is the pattern upon which you construct your body from energy. Consciousness creates form, not the other way around. It is upon this pattern of consciousness and thought that the energy is "stabilized" into "solid" matter. Your conscious mind produces thoughts, which are actually electromagnetic fields. The combination of these forms of energy creates the physical body, and this creation is an active and ongoing process. The body is reconstructed according to directions from your conscious mind, and directions are being given every second of every day. Therefore, your thoughts and beliefs determine whether you will be healthy or sickly.

Under certain conditions, you will yourself to be sick. If others fall sick around you, you may accept sickness as inevitable, or actually seek it, and your body complies with the unconscious wish. If you see yourself as sinful or unworthy, these thought patterns direct how your body will react and may produce illness as a form of punishment that you think you deserve. If you believe that aggressive feelings can be expressed only through violence and never in creative ways, while your ethical code precludes your acting out violence, then this internal conflict will eventually be turned back upon you. There are many scenarios in which our thoughts "turn against us" following our accepted core beliefs and direct our bodies in ways that we do not consciously intend. Our subconscious minds are very creative, and the cells always joyfully comply with the intent of the mind.

Even the vast majority of injuries are psychosomatically induced. Statistics show that ninety percent of all accidents occur to ten percent of the people. These are the folks known to be accident prone. Psychological studies have repeatedly revealed that these individuals have guilts and beliefs that render them self-destructive. They do not commit suicide. They just hurt pieces of themselves from time to time, breaking a leg here, chopping off a finger there. A study was done with truck drivers who had impeccable records for safety but had recently had an accident. A careful psychological interview with these drivers showed that on the particular day of their collisions, they were "accident prone." Something had occurred in their lives for which they felt accountable, such as a rare marital fight, an altercation with the boss, or an illness in the family for which, for some reason, the trucker blamed himself. The accident was each driver's way of obtaining punishment.

The second principle to be understood, and to which I have already referred, is that every cell in your body has memory, consciousness, intent, and the ability to communicate with other cells. The intent is primarily one of joyful cooperation with the conscious mind. Thus, the cells joyfully take instruction and produce the cellular response suggested by the conscious mind—as in the old people who made themselves younger. If the conscious or subconscious mind instructs your cells to remain "sick or injured" for whatever reason, then the cells will follow those directions, regardless of the efforts of your physician or your ego. It is important to understand that your conscious mind belongs to your spirit. It is the same mind you have had from your beginning and the one you will always have. When you incarnate, your conscious mind simply fuses with your brain and nervous system and uses that network to communicate with the body and with the outside world.

For these reasons, an injury such as Harry believes he sustained when his skull was crushed in 1784 was sufficient to cause his migraines. Similarly, illnesses and injuries sometimes fail to get well because the cells have been given instructions to the contrary.

When I used to try explaining psychosomatic disease to my patients, they would ask, "Is it in my mind, or do I really have something wrong with me?" My reply was always "Yes." I would try to explain that it didn't matter, that there really was no difference. Some of them got it; most did not. That's the way it is with the medical profession. Most doctors don't get it either, and most never will, because their training precludes their understanding. So they go on, trying to treat sick people as if they were machines in need of adjustment. Too many physicians are incapable of dealing with the spiritual aspect of humanity. They look for the easy explanation and the quick fix. It is the lay public, the informed patient, who must demand better of our M.D.'s, our chiropractors, dentists, homeopaths, and psychologists. The knowledge—and a lot of the know-how—is out there. As patients, we must force our doctors to change, force them to throw off the blinders and learn to be healers.

NEUROLOGICAL
DEVELOPMENT

I HAD BEEN IN PRACTICE only a few years when I met a man who later became one of my best friends. I was at a party and started talking with a gentleman who impressed me with his intelligence and honesty. Phil Kessler, I found out, was an optometrist. I had been taught in medical school that optometrists were minimally trained to fit glasses and little else. As a matter of fact, in the 1950s the AMA still classified them as cultists and did not consider them to be professionals.

As Phil and I became close friends, I began to inquire about his training, asking him how he could pretend to fit glasses properly when he was not allowed to use drugs to dilate the pupils? He explained that one could no more fit glasses with the muscles of accommodation paralyzed than tune the engine of an automobile with the motor shut off. Vision is a dynamic process involving the brain, he explained, and not a mechanical optical function within the eye. He informed me that optometrists are fully trained in ocular pathology and are the major source of referrals to the ophthalmologists. At that time, there were some 26,000 optometrists and only about 8,000 ophthalmologists in the country. It was obvious from the numbers alone that most people were going to optometrists for their visual problems. But in medical school, we were led to believe they were an unskilled and untrained minority.

I learned a lot from Phil. He was a good teacher and a good friend. Through him, I became aware of the Optometric Extension Program and the effectiveness of vision training. He also taught me much about how vision develops and how children develop neurologically. These new concepts—of which I had never heard so much as a hint during my medical training—sent me to the library. I was practicing then in Champaign, Illinois, and the entire University of Illinois library was available to me. For the next two years, I spent every spare moment reading books on educational psychology and neurological development. I am quite certain few doctors have read one book on either subject and certainly not the wide scope of works I hungrily devoured. It was exciting and fun!

As a result of this new-found knowledge, I joined Dr. Kessler in putting together a developmental program for children who had visual-motor-perceptual problems. The program was based upon tried-and-true methods of therapy as taught in the Optometric Extension Program and built upon years of research done by numerous developmental psychologists. After we had been working together about a year, Phil and I went to Philadelphia to visit Glen Doman and Carl Delacato, who ran the Institute for the Achievement of Human Potential. The institute was established specifically for the treatment of brain injured and retarded children. There was a lot of talk about the institute in those days, and we wanted to see firsthand what they were doing. We were impressed with their program but felt it lacked the input of an optometrist at that time. Delacato was attempting to fill the gap, but his training was as an educator, not an optometrist. We felt he was in over his head, and I am certain Delacato would have admitted it had we discussed the problem with him. But the therapy at the institute worked, and it was based upon the same principles that I had learned reading developmental psychology and neurology in the University of

Illinois library. In fact, it was identical to the principles taught by the Optometric Extension Program.

Phil and I also developed an environmental program for parents to use with their normal infants and babies. The elements of the program were based on the premise that unless an infant is allowed to develop his or her movement patterns in a free and appropriate manner, the brain and nervous system will not develop normally. To some degree, large or small, in one way or another, if the child is prevented from doing this, the child will be handicapped.

Probably the most dramatic example from my own practice involved Carl, who was born to a young couple completing their Ph.D. degrees at the university. I outlined to the parents what they should do, such as placing Carl on the floor on his belly. (The details will be given later in the chapter.) They both appeared to be very interested and readily agreed. Carl was a very unhappy baby who constantly screamed at the top of his lungs. In retrospect, my judgment is that he probably was minimally brain injured, but it was not evident at the time. Every single time Carl was brought to the office, he screamed. You could hear him out in the hallway before he entered the waiting room. His mother and I would converse, yelling at each other, trying to be heard over Carl's screeching. I would inquire as to how he was doing developmentally, and she would assure me that everything was progressing normally.

When Carl was three, his mother came to the office alone. Her eyes were swollen and red from crying. I asked what was wrong. Through her tears, she told me they had taken Carl to three different board-certified pediatricians who had independently given them the same diagnosis. All three had told them that Carl was hopelessly mentally retarded and "homicidal" and should be placed in a mental hospital immediately.

I couldn't believe what I was hearing. I asked her the basis for these seemingly outlandish diagnoses. Come on, a three-year-old child diagnosed as homicidal? She replied that Carl had never spo-

CONFESSIONS OF A HEALER

ken a single word, not even "ma-ma" or "da-da." As far as the homicidal part was concerned, he had injured several children by hitting
them on the head with various toys. I knew immediately that they
had never put the child on the floor.

"Kit, you've lied to me! You never put Carl on the floor, did
you?" I was angry, really angry.

Her mouth sagged and she began to stammer.

"Well, did you?"

"No," she confessed, "I carried him."

"By not following my directions, and carrying him all the time,
it looks as though you have retarded his development. Unless you just
want to get him off your hands, I suggest you start listening to me!"

She was sobbing at this point, swearing she did not want to
abandon the boy. She vowed that she and her husband would do anything and everything I suggested. I told her I could promise nothing
but since he was only three, he had a chance, providing they followed directions. I instructed her to make him a corset to wear over
his clothing, with straps going over his shoulders so it could not be
pulled down. She was to attach a metal ring to the corset over his tail
bone. I told her to get two large screw eyes and screw one into the
back of the heel of each shoe. Then a rope was to be strung from the
screw eye in one heel, up through the ring at his tail bone and down
to the other heel. The rope was to be of such a length that, when he
straightened out one leg, the other would be drawn up to his butt.
With this harness in place, Carl would be unable to stand, since he
wasn't well enough coordinated to balance on one leg. The harness
was similar to that I had observed being used when Phil and I
visited Glen Doman's institute.

With the boy unable to be upright, she was to get down on
the floor and play with him, helping him to creep on hands and
knees. Kit agreed to keep Carl in the harness twenty-four hours a day.
What's more, if he pulled himself upright using the furniture, she
was to place him back on the floor on all fours. Being in a vertical

position before the child has developed in the horizontal plane retards certain elements of neurological development. So it was essential for Carl to be kept on his hands and knees and not allowed to stand or walk. I gave her an appointment to return in four weeks with Carl to allow me to evaluate his progress.

The month passed, and Kit did not keep the appointment. I called her asking what was going on. She said Carl had been unable to creep when first placed on the floor. I would have been surprised if he *had* been able to creep. She said he had just barely started creeping on hands and knees and had finally stopped screaming. She swore she kept him in the harness all day and removed it only when she gave him his bath. I instructed her to bring him to the office in another month or I'd send the police for them. She knew I was not kidding.

At the end of his second month on the floor, Kit brought Carl to my office. When I entered the exam room, he was sitting quietly on her lap in his harness, and, for the first time I'd seen him since he'd been born, he was not screaming.

"Well, Carl, how are you?" I asked.

"I'm just fine, Dr. Bonnett. How are you?" He spoke clearly, in well-articulated language.

I was so surprised I nearly fell out of my chair. We all burst out laughing. From no speech to complete sentences in eight weeks was a bit more than I expected. Kit went on to say he had started saying single words about three weeks before and then "language started tumbling out." I referred Carl to Dr. Kessler, who placed him on a full vision training program, and continued to follow up with the boy's development.

Some years after I moved to Ohio, I received a letter from a teacher who had been aware of Carl's problem. She taught Carl in kindergarten and at the end of the year promoted him to first grade. One week into first, the teacher called his parents telling them he did not belong there. She moved him on to second grade. So it went through the years, skipping a number of grades. Enclosed in the letter was a newspaper clipping stating that Carl had just won a National Science Foundation Fellowship to MIT at the age of fifteen.

This young genius would have lived a life of frustration in a mental hospital had he not been allowed to develop his visual-motor-perceptive skills. I've often wondered how the three pediatricians would explain the outcome.

Because of its importance in the development and well-being of children, it seems that knowledge of neurological development should be required of anyone caring for the young. But traditionally, little if anything has been taught in medical schools or residency training about child development. The doctor is told that the average child sits up at six months and begins to talk and walk at one year. That's about it. The information is all readily available; it just isn't in medical literature and thus it's read by precious few practicing physicians.

When an infant is born, the most acutely developed sense is the sense of touch. The most sensitive areas for touch are the lips and tongue. The reason for this is that newborn animals need to find the nipple to suckle and survive. Their mothers can't pick them up and place their mouths to the nipple as can humans. Still, this locating reflex is present in human infants and can be readily demonstrated by touching the baby's cheek and observing him turn his head to suck on your finger.

The least developed sense at birth is the sense of sight. The newborn is, in order of decreasing skill, a tactile, kinesthetic, auditory, visual creature. Kinesthesia is the ability to feel movement and sense the location and position of the body and limbs. By the time a child is six, if everything has gone well, the child will have reversed the order, becoming a visual, auditory, kinesthetic, tactile person. Let's discuss in brief how all this evolves.

The newborn sees little other than moving patterns of light. He feels a lot with his lips and tongue, primarily the nipple and bot-

tle or breast. He soon discovers there is another area of skin, far easier to move about than his mouth, and almost as sensitive. That skin
is on his index finger and thumb. At the same time, his brain is
being bombarded by nerve impulses as light flickers on the retina of
his eyes. Before long, in the process of waving his hands, he begins to
get the idea that moving his hands causes the pattern of light to
change in his visual world. What is happening out in space is responsible for the light pattern he sees. It is not something occurring in
his eyeballs—it is "out there."

This association of activity in space with the stimulus taking
place in his eyes is the beginning of vision. As he lies on his belly, the
movements of his arms and legs, which are at first spontaneous and
non-directed, start to become programmed as he learns that certain
motions allow him to move and others do not. As he moves and
crawls, he observes changes in the light pattern.

The eye does not work like a reflex camera. When you look
at a horse, there is not an image of a horse cast upside down on the
retina of your eye, as we all were taught. For every point of light in
space, there is a pattern of light cast on the retina. We have to learn
to interpret what that pattern represents. We do this by feeling,
touching, reaching, and manipulating what we see with our fingers
until a tactile-motor-visual match is constructed in our brains. Allvar
Gullstrand, a Swedish physician, received the Nobel Prize in medicine in 1911 for his work proving that the eye does not work like a
camera. Here we are, eighty-some years later, still going on a false
and outdated premise. In fact, an article in a recent issue of *National
Geographic* indicated the eye worked like a camera. Humankind
seems opposed to adopting new ideas and abandoning outdated and
inaccurate ones.

From the moment a child is born to about nine months, she
is monocular. That is, her eyes see more or less independently. They
may appear straight, but they do not work in concert. Binocularity
develops by her creeping on all fours, starting in about the ninth

month. By crawling and creeping the infant develops a sense of "center" within her body and a sense of laterality, or of what is off center. Later, she learns to call it left and right. When she starts getting up on her hands and knees at about five months, her center becomes more important, for if she gets off center, she falls. All this is critical to her visual development. Without the concepts of center, left and right, top and bottom, front and back, firmly established within her body, she cannot project these concepts into space and apply them to what she sees. We create our visual world and literally project it into space, almost like a movie projector. Thus, we do not experience sight as occurring in our eyes as we do taste within our mouths. The image, which is a function of the brain, not the eye, is projected in space, and the accuracy with which this is done depends upon the concept of space within ourselves. To repeat, the only way this is achieved is through the process of crawling, creeping and feeling our way about during those early critical months.

As the child experiments on hands and knees he soon learns to sit up—all by himself. Propping a child in a sitting position until he learns to balance is not sitting. Watching your baby get into a sitting position, with no help from anyone, is a genuine thrill. That's sitting! Sitting adds new dimensions to space for the infant. It adds front and back, and top and bottom, along the vertical axis of the body. Shortly thereafter, he will begin to creep on hands and knees. Creeping is critical to the total development of the neurological process. Children should creep at least three months before they start walking much. Even after the child is able to walk, it is a good idea to play with him on the floor, encouraging him to creep on hands and knees. Don't worry if your child continues to creep after he learns how to walk. I've never known anyone going to college creeping, but I've known a lot of kids who never made it to college because they didn't creep enough, or at all. It is through creeping that nerve pathways within the midbrain are formed which coordinate and fuse the movement of the eyes into a functional unit. This is the stage when early hand-eye coordination is developing rapidly.

Creeping involves the motor pattern of the arms and legs that is carried on into walking. This movement pattern is called "cross-pattern" movement. The left hand and right leg move forward more or less at the same time; then the right hand and left leg take their turn. Watch some person clumping down the street, his arms hanging stiffly at his sides. Chances are, he didn't creep much, if at all, and he may well have trouble reading.

If a child is placed in the vertical position by the use of walkers, bounce chairs, swings, and such, and is later taught to walk, thereby skipping the crawling and creeping phase, she will have problems. As with Carl, speech may be delayed. Often she will develop strabismus, or crossed eyes. Even more often, the vision of one eye will not develop—a condition called amblyopia, or lazy eye—or she may have problems reading.

A friend of mine was a professor in the College of Educational Administration at the University of Illinois. He spent years helping the Bolivian government set up an educational system. Before their revolution in the early 1950s, it had been a capital offense to teach an Indian to read. After the revolution, the new government wanted everyone to have a good education. My friend told me it was virtually impossible to teach the Indians to read much past the third-grade level. Moreover, the vast majority of them were obviously cross-eyed. Anthropologists had a theory that the crossed eyes were due to the extremely high altitude. La Paz, the capital of Bolivia, is at almost 12,000 feet elevation. It is the highest capital in the world. You land at the airport and the stewardess stands in the door of the plane with an oxygen mask on, saying, "Enjoy your stay in La Paz." But it is not the altitude that causes the people to be cross-eyed and to have difficulty reading. It is the custom of the Bolivian Indians to carry their babies in slings on the mothers' backs. They are never put on the floor or the ground to crawl and creep.

When the children are about eighteen months old, they are held by the hands and taught to walk, balancing them until they can totter about on their own. Here is a whole culture that handicaps itself from entering the modern world where reading is essential, by following an ancient custom of child rearing.

Reading involves recognizing shapes and patterns of words and letters. This is dependent upon the reader's being able to project the internal concepts of space into the environment. Without a right or left concept, a "b" looks the same as a "d." A top-bottom concept is necessary to distinguish a "b" and "p" as well as "d" and "q." These are all vertical lines with a bump on one side or the other, or one end or the other. Without the appropriate spatial concepts, bad, dad, pad, dap, qad, daq, pag and gap all become confused with each other. Words also sometimes become reversed, like "saw" and "was" or "on" and "no." Remember when you were in first grade and Billie was asked to read aloud? He read "Jane was the dog" and everyone laughed. Billie simply hadn't had sufficient time creeping on hands and knees. When we read a word such as "confusing," we recognize it largely by its shape. We see the "c" at the beginning, the letter sticking up near the middle with the crook, and the one hanging down at the end. Once we know the word, length and shape are more important than letter content. The vast majority of dyslexic cases are due to conceptual distortions of space caused by insufficient time spent crawling and creeping in the critical first year of life.

I have said that the infant is largely a creature of touch and movement who has to train his visual apparatus, the eye and the brain, to substitute for these functions. He sees an object and at the same time reaches for it. He learns to place it in space, whether it is right or left of center. Is it too far to reach, or does he have to creep some distance in order to touch it? Does he creep a little way or a long way? In this process, he learns to gauge distance. He feels the object. Is it smooth or rough to touch? He learns to recognize the visual patterns associated with the various textures. Early on, he does not always trust the validity of the information received from his hand and eyes, so what does he do? He goes back to the gold standard, that best and most reliable part of himself with which he started. He puts the object in his mouth. His lips and tongue tell him for sure whether it is smooth or rough, and all the variations between. Sigmund Freud spoke of this being the oral stage of gratification. This was pure speculation based upon an invalid premise that all early activities stem from oral gratification. Even now, as an adult, when you do not trust your eyes you probably don't go so far as to put the object in your mouth, but you reinforce your vision with touch. Remember the last time you had to touch a piece of leather or cloth to determine if your visual impression was correct?

By the age of six years, the child should have become a visual person, for she will learn primarily through her sense of sight. In first grade, a large number of children have trouble seeing the blackboard. When their visual acuity is checked, they *appear* to be nearsighted. A long time ago, researchers followed a bunch of these kids for a year, but did nothing to treat their visual problems. At the end of the year, the children were reexamined. A third were no more "nearsighted" than at the first examination, a third were a bit worse, and the final third had normal vision.

Another study was done in which the children, regardless of how their vision tested, were given a mild prescription for glasses which would enlarge things a bit. They were fit with glasses with about a half diopter of plus, just the opposite of what they appeared to require. These kids were rechecked after a year of wearing the glasses and almost all of them had normal vision! Some of them needed to wear the glasses a bit longer, but basically they were OK. They were neither far- nor nearsighted.

Being far- or nearsighted is not the result of a long or short eyeball. That kind of reasoning goes back to the false concept that the eye works like a camera, and that idea was disproved in 1911. Whether one is far- or nearsighted is a matter of how one perceives space. Monkeys can be made nearsighted by placing them in cages where they are never allowed to look at anything farther away than a foot or two.

What happens to most children is they are taken to an M.D., who tests their vision, does not understand visual development, and, finding them "nearsighted," prescribes minus lenses for them. The glasses make things sharper but smaller, like looking through the wrong end of a pair of field glasses. Within a year, the children are more myopic, so they get stronger glasses and so on. By the time they are in high school, they have fully retreated into myopia and are wearing contacts or lenses thick as the bottoms of pop bottles.

When I started school, like a lot of other kids, I was having trouble seeing the blackboard clearly. My mother took me to an old optometrist by the name of Dr. Sheib. He examined me and gave me a mild farsighted prescription. God bless him. I wore my glasses two years and then we went to visit relatives in Kansas. My Uncle Porter was a renowned obstetrician. He delivered me. He noticed I was wearing glasses and demanded to know why and who had prescribed them. When he forced my mother to admit that she had taken me to an optometrist, he threw up his hands in disgust, mumbled something about quacks, snatched the glasses off my face, broke them, and threw them into the trash. My poor uncle, in the ignorance that went along with being a physician, was a self-proclaimed authority on everything. Thanks to Dr. Sheib and the two years I did wear my plus prescription, I ended up OK.

So into what kind of physical environment should you place your baby? Freedom to move is the key, so, as I instructed Kit and her husband, a newborn baby should spend a great deal of time on the floor on his stomach. The house should be warm enough at floor level so it is right for the infant. The hands and feet should be bare in order for the baby to get a grip on the floor.

The baby should be kept there all day, and his parents should get on the floor to play with and love the child. They can, of course, pick him up to change diapers, feed him, love him, and rock him, but then they should return him to the floor on his belly.

To add further sensory input, I told my patients to play the radio for auditory stimulation. Blinking colored lights were to be strung along the baseboard on one wall. On other walls, cutouts of circles, squares and triangles made of colored paper were to be pasted. Several balls and blocks should be scattered on the floor just out of the baby's reach.

Occasionally, I told my patients to clap their hands or crash pots and pans together to accustom their infants to loud noises and help them overcome the startle reflex. They were to brush the palms of the baby's hands and soles of her feet with a fingernail brush several times a day.

The environment was to include a lot of loving, cuddling, talking, singing, and reading. These are essential for the emotional and spiritual development of the infant. All kids who are really loved receive these things. It is the sensory stimulation that is usually lacking—not through intent, but through ignorance of its need. It is amazing to see kids develop in this kind of surroundings, when they are placed on the floor and allowed to develop their visual-motor-perceptual skills. They are the brightest, smartest, most alert kids imaginable.

There is a practice these days that is so common and so harmful to the normal development of children that I must make special emphasis of it. I'm talking about the widespread use of bounce chairs, swings, walkers and other pieces of equipment designed to keep the infant in one spot, out from under foot. These baby-sitting contraptions cause problems in neurological development and, I'm tempted to say, even mental retardation. This may sound overly dramatic, but it is not.

Remember Carl, and the Indian kids in Bolivia? Their only problem was being carried rather than being given the opportunity to crawl and creep. There is no difference whether the kid is in a sling on the mother's back or sitting in a bounce chair or swing. For some reason, if an infant is placed upright in the vertical position before he has fully developed in the horizontal axis, gravity interferes with the nerve pathways in the brain and he will sustain retardation of his neurological development. Since we know the physical body is an electromagnetic field, this should not be too surprising. It is far more common to develop visual and reading difficulties, as do the Indians, than speech retardation. Carl had other problems besides his speech. When Dr. Kessler started working with him, he had the visual development of a one-year-old baby, and Carl was three.

So please, please, please don't put your baby in some sort of contraption. Put the kid on the floor on his stomach where he belongs. If you have one of these pieces of equipment, burn the damned thing. I don't care if grandmother did give it to him or how much it cost.

It was cold in Kansas the fall and winter of 1925. We lived in a drafty old house, so my dad made me a playpen using a huge packing crate. He lined it with an old quilt so I'd be warm and would not bump and scrape myself. I remember it was in a bay window on the south side of the house, right under a big Boston fern. It was a very nice playpen but, like all playpens, it gave me something to grab onto, so I could stand up. There wasn't much room for me to creep, either.

I need to explain that my conscious memory goes back to when I was only five or six weeks old. I documented this with my parents by recalling and relating incidents which they had forgotten and never visited about. I don't remember at what age I began to stand, but I do remember clearly teaching myself to walk by the age of eight months. Standing in my pen, I would walk around and around, holding onto the edge. Looking about the room was a lot more fun than being in the bottom of the box where I could see nothing except beige quilt. I clearly remember one day getting the idea of walking across the box. I could take two steps and lunge and usually grab the other side without falling. It was great fun and I practiced until I was good at it, long before I should have been. Like the Bolivian Indians, I had skipped the creeping phase of my development. I did not become cross-eyed. I was lucky. A severe illness intervened which, in a roundabout way, saved the day.

When we moved to Urbana, Illinois, I had just turned three. Within a month or two, I became severely ill with pneumonia. In 1928 there were no antibiotics. If you got sick you either lived or died with no real help from the doctor. He did what he could and gave me cough syrup and a gray tablet containing iodine to thin the mucus, and that was about it. I was placed in the hospital and lay there for over a week in a steam tent with my temperature going as high as 106.5. I recall overhearing the doctor tell the nurse that if my temperature went any higher, I would probably die. I didn't die, but I did suffer some minimal brain injury due to the fever. When I was able to go home, I couldn't walk!

I remember sitting in a little child-size rocking chair looking at my legs, wondering how to make them work. I could stand, but for the life of me I had no idea how to walk. I'd try and I'd fall. My mother didn't believe me and the doctor said it was because I was too weak. But I knew better, and I was scared. I began playing on the floor, creeping about and, in a couple of weeks, I was up walking again.

Now, I still had my original problem—that of not having sufficient creeping time as a result of walking prematurely. Several months later, we went to visit relatives, and I returned home with a brown and white puppy. My puppy saved me. For months, I played with Brownie, creeping all over the house, for hours on end. I even pretended I was a dog. I remember playing dog all winter. Eventually, I got my midbrain fairly well programmed. I did not end up with motor problems with my eyes, but I had some difficulty with right-left discrimination. I remember printing letters backward for quite a while. I just missed being dyslexic. All in all, I lucked out, through no help from anyone other than Brownie and Dr. Sheib. What I hope this story illustrates is how easily problems can develop. My guess is the majority of infants are dumped into a playpen or some other contraption in front of the TV and left there while their mothers or baby-sitters do what they want. No wonder there are so many dyslexics and other kids who have difficulty learning to read.

Dr. Kessler and I worked together for five or six years, until his untimely death. During that period, we managed to get twenty-two or twenty-three children out of retarded and special education classes into regular schools, where they made excellent grades. As a result, I came under attack by the county medical society—primarily the ophthalmologists. I wasn't surprised, for the doctors were following an age-old historical pattern of opposing anything not fitting into their belief system. The physicians and ophthalmologists in particular circulated false rumors about Phil and me. One was that we were giving written guarantees to parents that we would cure their kids. We also heard reports that we were charging untold thousands of dollars for our work. I figured up one time how much income I had lost working with these children and their parents. It turned out to be quite a chunk of money. I could never bring myself to charge for all the hours I spent. For a few of the cases, we charged nothing; the parents just didn't have any money. Finally, in an attempt to force me out of the county medical society, the ophthalmologists charged me with unethical conduct for working and consulting with a "cultist." It was true. I was working with an optometrist.

The interesting thing was that one of the clinics in the community had three ophthalmologists on its staff who were leading the charge against me. It had two optometrists on its staff, so the doctors there were working with "cultists," too. If I was unethical, then every doctor at the clinic in Champaign was equally unethical. If it hadn't been so serious, it would have been funny. In the 1950s a doctor had to be a member of the AMA in order to be on the staff of a hospital. If they had succeeded, I would have been in big trouble. But I did not give up, and eventually the charges all were dropped.

The problems and hostility we were facing fell within the lines of probability. There were other lines of probability; one was that Phil's and my work could have been accepted and applauded. We were fully aware at the outset that this was not likely. Doing something different, even if what you do is right, is often difficult. If we had not tried and accomplished what we did, there would be twenty more people in the world living handicapped or retarded. If we had feared being different, Carl would never have gone to MIT.

Dr. Kessler and I had a lot of success in the five or six years during which we worked together. One eight-year-old boy in my practice was having a terrible time reading and was cutting up in school. The teacher had already sent him to the psychologist, with no improvement. The parents finally brought him to me. On examination, I asked him to look at my finger and follow it with his eyes as I moved it about. He could not do it. Watching his eye movement, I noticed his eyes would follow for a second and then go shooting off to the side. Then he would fix on my finger for a moment only to shoot off to the side again. In vision, we speak of reaching, grasping, manipulating, and releasing an object in the same way we refer to handling an object with our hands. I asked the boy if he lost his place a lot when he was reading. He said he did and that the words jumped around all the time. Nobody can read when his eyes behave in such a manner. I asked his mother how much time he had spent creeping when he was small. She replied she could not remember him ever creeping. They had used a playpen and he started pulling up, standing, and walking very early. She had been pleased, for she had heard this meant he was very bright. Imagine the shock and disappointment to find your "bright" child in the remedial reading section at school. I referred them to Phil, who convinced them to put the lad on a full vision training program. After about six months of intensive work at home, he was in a normal reading class making straight A's.

The fact that the school system was disturbed by our work and success did surprise us a bit. I suspect the teachers knew little more than the doctors about child development and educational psychology. In any case, we were upsetting the system. Retarded or handicapped kids were supposed to stay that way. It was OK to *try* to help them, but never, never should one cure them. There were budgets to consider. Money was appropriated according to the number of children in each category. Being forced to reassign them to regular classes threw the budgets all off. Then there was the embarrassment of it all. After dealing with the parents and establishing that their kids were dyslexic and could not read, to have some GP and an optometrist work with them a few months and make the children normal was too much to accept.

We all succumb to negative pressure at one time or another. There have been times I did not have the energy to do what I knew was best. I didn't have the energy to present the alternative plan, answer all the questions, defend the position, and listen to all the doubts. It was just easier to give the antibiotic prescription for the cold than to explain once more that it would do no good.

Those of us who have listened to the different drummer all our lives become tired and discouraged. Invariably, upon being offered an alternative therapy, most patients go off to seek a second opinion. Chances are that the other doctor, steeped in conventional wisdom and not having a clue about what has been proposed, is not really in a position to give a valid second opinion. For a second opinion to be of any real value the physician should at least be familiar with the subject or the method, even if she does not choose to practice that way herself. Thus, many of my patients either would not return, convinced I was too unconventional, or would return untrusting and skeptical. In the real world, you can't afford to turn all your patients away. Doctors have to pay their bills, too.

I have spoken of the Optometric Extension Program. It deserves further comment. As I recall, it began about 1928 after its founder, Dr. M. A. Skeffington, discovered a person's sight in both eyes might appear to be fused but is often fused only by the act of fixation on the visual target. The technical term for this condition is "phoria." Glasses which were fit to each eye individually could not be worn with comfort when a patient suffering a phoria put them on and started looking with both eyes at once. Dr. Skeffington visited the Gesell Institute, which was devoted to studying child development. He asked what they knew about how children learned to see. They admitted they knew little beyond the fact that infants did not see as adults see.

Skeffington related his findings, which prompted the institute to launch a study of visual development in children. It brought some optometrists on staff, George Crow for one, and began to do research. The result was the writing of a book in the early 1940s on the development of vision in infancy and childhood. The institute was immediately criticized by the medical profession—because its staff included optometrists.

Information was being discovered that was so important to the practicing optometrist that Skeffington decided his role should be to distribute this material to the optometrists in the field. He founded the OEP, whose journal is published on a regular basis. It also holds training workshops for optometrists throughout the country.

These are the doctors, these optometrists, who are qualified to straighten out your kid's crossed eyes. These are the doctors to whom you should take your child if she holds her head a couple of inches from her coloring book or is having trouble in school. The psychologist may be needed somewhere along the way, but before you and the teacher decide that your kid's mind is screwed up, it makes sense to find out if she can see and process information visually.

If your child has a stick run into his eyeball, develops an infection, or has a tumor in his eye, then, by all means, see a medical doctor. If Grandma develops a cataract, the doctor can fix that, but then take her to an optometrist to fit her glasses. Anyone who has a visual problem should see an optometrist, and if there is one who is a member of the OEP, choose that one.

It is of critical importance for every parent to understand how an infant develops and to place the child in an environment that will be helpful to ensure his or her success. It is also imperative that medical schools, as well as pediatric and family practice residency programs, teach the same material. If we are to compete in the modern world, we must equip children to do this through education, and if our children are to be educated, they must be neurologically capable of being educated in the first place. We would not build Olympic swimming pools for a generation of children with no arms or legs. Unfortunately, this is analogous to the present situation, when a large percentage of kids leave high school unable to read past the third- or fourth-grade level. As individuals and as a nation, there is much to accomplish by thinking outside of convention.

SIX

HEART ATTACK

The Preventable Disease

H EART DISEASE is such a feared and widespread illness
that I want to put a lot of information about it in a neat little pile here in this chapter. Diseases of the heart and vascular system account for 42 percent of all deaths in the
United States. Therefore, when we discuss this subject we are considering a form of death that will affect nearly everyone in some way,
whether it is yourself or a close relative whom a heart attack strikes.

In the old days, when I started practice over forty years ago,
if a man went to the doctor having heart pain, there was little to do
other than prescribe nitroglycerin and advise the patient to stop
smoking and refrain from physical exertion. In those days, there
weren't even any effective drugs to treat high blood pressure.
Doctors would follow their patients for weeks, sometimes years, waiting for the inevitable heart attack. Some physicians tested the
patients' cholesterol levels, but since nothing was known about treating high cholesterol anyway, it didn't really make sense to put the
patient to the expense of running the periodic tests. Until fairly
recently, a cholesterol level of 250 or 300 was considered to be within
normal range. I never felt those were normal values. True, they were
what were found in a great many Americans, but there is a big differ-

ence between a laboratory norm and a physiologic normal. It would be like saying that dental caries is normal just because most people have fillings or cavities in their teeth. Ideally, your cholesterol level should be below 220.

One day, I read a research paper by Hans Selye, a professor of physiology at the University of Montreal. Working in his laboratory with white rats, Selye had discovered some exciting and astounding things. He anesthetized a white rat, opened its chest cavity, and exposed the heart. Then, using a surgical ligature, he took a stitch in the front of the heart, tying off the main coronary artery, which supplies most of the blood to the entire front and lateral portion of the left ventricle. He did this to a large bunch of rats. As you might expect, with the blood supply to the heart muscle tied off, the rats all died of massive heart attacks. Some did not live to have their chests sewn up, and those that did survive the surgery died within a day or two. It is important for you to remember that *all* the rats died.

Next, he took another group of rats and performed the exact same surgical procedure, only this bunch of rats had been given large amounts of potassium chloride before the surgery and continued to receive the potassium after the artery was ligated. Surprise! Not a single rat died! After a few days, he killed the rats and did autopsies on them. First, he made sure the stitch had indeed blocked the artery. It had. Then he examined the heart muscle. Some of the rats showed no sign whatsoever of any damage to the heart muscle. Most of them had patches of dead and dying muscle, but not sufficient to cause the rats to die. Selye found magnesium chloride was just as effective as potassium chloride. A few other salts, such as ammonium chloride, had some protective effect, but not to the same degree as the potassium and magnesium salts.

I had never heard anything like this. At the time, I had a patient in the hospital with an impending heart attack, so the information was very timely. I picked up the telephone, called the University of Montreal, and asked to speak with Dr. Selye. His secretary answered. I explained that I did not know the doctor but had read his article and wanted to visit with him about it. She said he was sitting beside her, was not doing anything at the moment, and would be delighted to talk.

I explained to Dr. Selye that I was a physician and wished to know how much potassium he had given to the rats. He reminded me he was a research scientist and did not treat people. I replied I had no rats in my practice, at least no four-legged ones, and urged him to give me the information I sought. Together, we figured out an equivalent dose that could be applied to humans.

The next day, I prescribed potassium and ammonium chloride tablets for my patient. By the following morning he was pain free. This sort of thing, calling up a doctor and trying an untested treatment, could not be done today. But that was forty years ago. Now there are too many restrictions and the ever-present danger of lawsuits. Things have changed. Anyway, my patient left the hospital in a couple of days. I followed him for about a year. He continued to take his potassium chloride and to stay on the low-salt diet I had prescribed. When he moved from the community, he was still free of angina and had not had a myocardial infarct.

Another aspect of Selye's work involved stress-induced heart attacks. Again using white rats, he devised a method to produce maximum stress in the animals. Rats can't float. If they are placed in a vat of water, they must swim or drown. It is a good method of producing stress through total physical exhaustion. Selye placed a group of rats into a vat of water and, just when their heads were going under, would rescue them and allow them to recover. A few of the rats would die from exhaustion and stress. On examination, they would be found to have sustained a heart attack.

Selye experimented to find what might produce an additive effect to the stress of swimming. He found that an injection of certain adrenal hormones dramatically increased the incidence of heart attack. The adrenal hormones were ones the body ordinarily produces during stress. Next, he tried table salt. Rats given a diet high in sodium had a very high death rate from heart attack when they were stressed. If he added an injection of the adrenal hormone to the high-salt diet, nearly all the rats died of massive infarcts.

Keep in mind that none of these animals had anything wrong with their coronary arteries. They were healthy young rats. The only thing done to them was to place them on a high-sodium diet and increase their stress, with or without the injections of the adrenal steroids. Now, we're talking exciting stuff! We're talking medical revolution! This demands a complete reevaluation of how the entire medical profession views heart attacks, from their cause to their treatment. Brace yourself for a real upheaval. As chairman Mao said, "A revolution is not a tea party." The problem was that the revolution never began. The medical profession, if they ever heard of Selye's work, ignored it and remained dedicated to the mechanical theory of heart attacks. Rather than thinking of heart disease as a cellular disease caused by stress and electrolyte imbalance as Selye had shown, the surgeons continued to attack the arteries.

I began with enthusiasm to approach patients in my practice from this new electrochemical viewpoint. I continued to preach the dangers of smoking. I stressed the importance of avoiding saturated fats, continued to treat high blood pressure vigorously and prescribed vitamin-mineral supplements. But in addition to these, I started prescribing potassium chloride supplements. Then, I really attacked the problem of sodium in the diet. My patients were not to use salt in cooking or in seasoning food at the table. I urged them to avoid foods obviously salty, such as chips, pickles, olives, hot dogs, canned meat, and canned vegetables. They were encouraged to eat fresh vegetables and meat, seasoning the food with herbs and spices other than salt.

Minimal elevations of blood pressure were not ignored, as my colleagues were prone to do. If the systolic blood pressure did not come down with the low salt diet, I prescribed medicine. I avoided the use of diuretics, unless I could bring the blood pressure down in no other way. Diuretics, or "water pills," were the most commonly prescribed drugs to treat hypertension in those days. But I knew diuretics damaged the sodium-potassium ATPase pump within the cell wall, causing an increase of sodium retained within the cell and a proportionate decrease of potassium remaining inside the cell. The ATPase pump is a mechanism within the cell wall that regulates the critical balance of potassium in the cell by pumping sodium out of the heart cell after each contraction. True, diuretics lower blood pressure by increasing the ability of the kidney to excrete salt, but I was convinced the damage to the ATPase pump and the concomitant loss of intracellular potassium would increase the risk of heart attack and death, thereby outweighing any benefit from lowering the blood pressure. Besides, there were a lot of other good drugs to treat high blood pressure. Years later, someone published a research paper proving I had been right.

The result of this different approach was that I rarely had patients develop heart attacks if they had been coming to me for any period of time. The heart attack patients I did see were, by and large, new patients and individuals who came to the emergency room having no doctor. Moreover, new patients I did treat for heart attacks rarely had another while following my program of medical management.

In 1970, I learned that a Mexican physician, Demetrio Sodi-Pallares, who was an expert in the field of electrocardiography, had just published a paper on his treatment of 100 patients with myocardial infarctions. His treatment was totally new and unlike anything used before. For patients under his treatment, he reported only a five percent mortality! This was at a time when the best coronary treatment centers around the world were experiencing a fifteen to twenty percent mortality using standard methods. A five percent mortality rate was unbelievable.

Dr. Sodi's treatment centered on the concept that a heart attack was basically an electrochemical event caused by an imbalance of sodium and potassium within the cell in the presence of stress. This is what Selye had proposed in his article from his work on rats, and now Dr. Sodi was using the method on people. These circumstances of a high sodium diet and stress were made worse by a decrease in oxygen due to coronary atherosclerosis. His treatment consisted of several elements:

1. *Very low sodium diet (500 milligrams a day)*
2. *Intravenous insulin*
3. *Continuous intravenous hypertonic glucose solution*
4. *Potassium supplements to ensure a blood level above 4.6 milliequivalents per liter*
5. *Sufficient water to ensure a moderately high urine volume*

One thing his treatment hinged upon was the administration of insulin to everyone, whether the patient was diabetic or not. Glucose was given to keep him or her from developing a low blood sugar. Research done by a French physician named Labroit had proved heart muscle to be dependent on insulin in order to burn sugar. Skeletal muscle does not need insulin, but heart muscle does.

The purpose of the treatment was to bathe the heart muscle with blood low in sodium and high in potassium, insulin, and glucose. Doing so made the work of the sodium-potassium ATPase pump easier. We all live or die depending on the efficiency of the ATPase pump, because every cell in the body, not just heart cells, regulates its sodium and potassium concentrations with this mechanism. The results of this treatment program are dramatic.

As is standard procedure, other doctors rushed to see if Sodi's results could be duplicated. Soon after Dr. Sodi's paper was published, a group of British physicians published a paper claiming they had been unable to duplicate his results. They stated that the treatment did no harm but did no good, either. If one reads the two papers there is no comparison. The British did not give insulin, except to diabetics, saying that for the rest of the patients in the study it was unnecessary. Nor did they give the concentrated glucose solution, arguing that the patients could drink and, therefore, did not need an intravenous—certainly not a 20-percent solution. Potassium was not administered, either, unless the serum potassium was below 3.5 meq—far below the level recommended by Dr. Sodi. Last, the British physicians did not prescribe a low sodium diet (though they did remove the salt packets from the patients' trays). In short, they did not do one single, solitary thing outlined in Dr. Sodi's protocol. Yet they claimed to have duplicated his work. Their paper was totally misleading.

Whom do you suppose the medical profession believed? Right. Why would anyone believe a Mexican working in Mexico, when his findings appeared to contradict those of the American and English physicians?

Well, I believed. I went to visit Dr. Sodi in Mexico City. I spent about ten days with him and his associates and found them to be extremely intelligent, well-read, honest, sincere individuals—to a man. They were dedicated and superb scientists.

The second or third day I was there, Dr. Sodi handed me a very thick manila envelope. It was unopened and still sealed with sealing wax imprinted with his personal crest. It had been addressed and mailed to one of the leading cardiology journals in the States. Over the original address was pasted a mailing label returning it to Dr. Sodi. He told me that after his original article had been published, he had been urged to publish another article with more patients to document further the effectiveness of his treatment. The manila envelope contained such a paper, describing his treatment of an additional 250 patients. It represented over three years' work for Dr. Sodi and his group of cardiologists. The results had been identical with the first—a five percent mortality.

Then he handed me a letter from the publisher to whom he had mailed the article. The publisher had not so much as looked at the article. It had been returned unopened, in the original envelope, sealed with sealing wax. In the rejection letter, the publisher stated that the article did not meet the standards acceptable for the journal. He went on to say that if Dr. Sodi wished to rewrite and resubmit it, they would be happy to consider it for publication. I got sick to my stomach as I sat there in the presence of this fine physician and his associates, all of whom had been so crudely insulted.

"Why would he do such a thing? They didn't even open the envelope! All I've heard is 'send us more documentation.' So I wrote another article, and now this." He was angry and hurt.

All I could do was apologize for my arrogant countrymen. He had no problem with European publishers accepting his work, so I advised him to forget the United States and to give the Europeans the benefit of his knowledge, instead.

But Dr. Sodi's was the treatment program I used for the next seventeen years, until my retirement. My personal series of patients had a mortality rate of seven percent. But then, North Americans don't have as good a diet as do Mexicans, at least when it comes to surviving heart attacks. For one thing, Mexicans eat more beans and fruit and get more magnesium and potassium in their diet.

Years ago, before coronary artery bypass surgery, surgeons attempted to get more blood to the heart by implanting the internal mammary artery, which runs down the inside of the chest wall, directly into the heart muscle. I always thought it was a stupid and irrational thing to do, but the patients who had undergone the procedure reported less pain, greater tolerance to exercise, and all the other benefits that patients report who have bypass surgery today. A big midwestern clinic was doing these operations right and left with considerable success. Then a surgeon on its staff did an experiment. He operated on a series of people who were told they were to have an internal mammary implant, but instead he made an incision down the middle of their chests, split the breast bones, and sewed them up without so much as touching their hearts. This is known as a "sham procedure." These patients reported the same marvelous results. The great results had to be the effect of suggestion. But an internal mammary implant is certainly a dangerous and expensive "sugar pill."

When bypass surgery started to be performed, patients were told they would die without the operation, that it was the only thing available to save them. Many were rushed to the operating room almost before they had time to think. This approach is still being used by many cardiac surgeons to panic patients into having surgery. I believe the only excuse is that the surgeons have honestly convinced themselves that what they say is true.

Studies have been performed showing that coronary bypass surgery is of no benefit in reducing mortality, unless the main left artery is closed (or some equivalent combination of major branches are blocked at the point where they arise from the main one). Following coronary bypass, there is no decrease in the number of heart attacks, either, and patients live no longer with the surgery than they would have lived without it. The only benefit is decreased heart pain, and some of the patients would have lived longer *without* the surgery. How many of you would take a pill intended to decrease your pain knowing that two or three out of every 100 people taking the medicine drop dead after swallowing the first tablet? Two or three deaths out of 100 is the mortality of bypass surgery in the very best hospitals.

Whenever I watched autopsies of people who had died of heart attacks, the pathologist would invariably point out the coronary arteries clogged with fatty deposits. Obviously the arteries had not gotten that way over night. I'd ask, "Why today? Why did it happen now, as opposed to last week, or a month ago?" He would laugh, saying I was asking an impossible question.

Some years ago, I attended a meeting at which Dr. Robert Lown of Harvard was a speaker. He finished giving his paper and started to leave the podium. Suddenly, he returned, saying he was going to commandeer the time of the next speaker. He said he was a colleague and would forgive him.

Dr. Lown proceeded to tell of a research program he had been carrying on for a couple of years. It involved about 100 patients who had received coronary arteriography and were shown to have severe blockage in two or three major coronary arteries. They were all candidates for bypass surgery but, for reasons of their own, had refused the surgery. Instead, they had enrolled in a medical treatment program run by Dr. Lown and his associates. Each patient was placed on strict medical management consisting of a very low-salt diet, potassium supplements, and vitamins, and all were urged to stop smoking. Strict attention was paid to lowering their blood pressure if it was high. Dr. Lown had been following these patients for over a year and had fewer deaths and heart attacks among this group of patients than a similar group who had undergone surgery.

He went on to say that Harvard had placed a lot of pressure on him *not* to publish the results of the study. Harvard, as do all big medical centers, has many hundreds of thousands of dollars invested in equipment to do bypass surgery.

In my practice, I treated one lady with severe coronary artery disease. Mary's EKG showed a chronic injury pattern and with mild exercise on the treadmill, she had a three- or four-millimeter drop of her ST segments across her entire left ventricle. All this means is that she was in deep trouble. Any slight exertion produced chest pain. She had a systolic blood pressure of 180, and her cholesterol was elevated. She had experienced several bouts of mild heart failure. Her previous doctor had her on a diuretic and a standard dose of digoxin—another drug that damages the sodium-potassium pump. In addition, she was a mild diabetic with a fasting blood sugar of 140. Her blood potassium was 3.5.

Mary did not want surgery. She had heard about me and wanted to try good medical management. The first thing I did was to stop her diuretic and the digoxin and place her on a 500-milligram sodium diet with a potassium supplement. I gave her a prescription for vitamins and encouraged her to reduce the saturated fat in her diet. In a matter of a week, her chest pain was all but gone and her systolic blood pressure was down to 150.

The second week, I repeated her EKG. It still showed some chronic injury in the lateral chest leads, so I convinced her to start small doses of insulin. Her mother was a diabetic, so giving herself an injection was no big deal. I put her on five units of Ultralente insulin every morning.

At the end of a month, she was totally pain free. Her systolic blood pressure was 138, the EKG was normal, and her cholesterol had dropped from 325 to 240. When I retired several years later, Mary was doing fine.

About a year after getting Mary squared away, her husband, who was going to an internist, was referred for coronary bypass surgery. She told me her husband had the identical problems she had—chest pain, heart failure, high blood pressure, diabetes, the works. The only difference was that he smoked two packs a day. The internist had told him to "watch his salt intake," but had not placed him on an actual diet. He had been placed on two different diuretics at the same time and was prescribed a double dose of digoxin. He was advised not to smoke. After a few months of this type of care, he was referred to an excellent surgeon for coronary bypass surgery.

Mary related that her husband had a massive heart attack and a cardiac arrest while undergoing surgery. A few hours later, coronary angiograms revealed the bypasses to be clotted, so he was taken back to surgery that night and the procedure was redone. Five weeks and $45,000 later, he was home.

Several months later, I asked Mary how he was doing. She laughed, stating he seemed to be doing all right. Then she added that the surgeon had placed him on a rigid low-salt, low saturated fat diet, much like hers. He had stopped the diuretic and digoxin and placed him on a potassium supplement. He had succeeded in getting her husband to stop smoking as well. She went on to speculate whether it was the surgery or the excellent medical management that was responsible for his seeming good health.

Unfortunately, over the next year, under the care of his original internist, he was told that the rigid salt-free diet was unnecessary. Eating more salt caused water retention, his feet swelled and he was restarted on the diuretic. Sometime later, after a mild bout of heart failure, he was placed on digoxin. Somewhere along the way, the potassium supplement was forgotten. After about six months, he suffered a heart attack and died at home.

One further observation. A friend of mine, Dr. Jim Dabney, once told me that the acupuncture points located down the exact center of the breast bone were points he used to relieve heart pain. Could the surgeon be giving the patient a permanent acupuncture treatment as he cuts through the center of the chest? Is that why bypass surgery relieves the pain, or is it just an expensive placebo?

Now surgeons often slip a balloon into the artery and blow it up, thereby compressing the fatty plaques, increasing the diameter of the hole in the artery. This is only another procedure based on the idea that heart attacks are caused solely by blocked coronary arteries. Nobody would argue with the assertion that getting more oxygen to the heart helps, but remember that Selye caused heart attacks in rats with normal coronary arteries.

Regardless of what you or the medical profession believe, nobody has the final answer. A fairly recent study was done in the eastern part of the country in which researchers asked a large group of men two questions. They asked if the men were happy and if they liked their jobs. According to the survey, if the men answered yes to both questions they were very unlikely to have a heart attack, regardless of their blood pressure, cholesterol, or anything else. The reason for this is that psychic intent is far more important when it comes to life and death, or health and illness, than are any of the various things a doctor may test you for. The man who likes his job and is happy is not looking to die from a heart attack or any other cause.

Certainly, clogged arteries do not help the situation. A decrease in blood flow to the heart muscle is a factor in the development of a heart attack. However, anyone who has read other literature or looked beyond his or her nose must admit that the nutritional, electrolyte, psycho-social, and spiritual conditions that are present must be of at least equal importance. Why does it have to be only one thing or another exclusively? Why must doctors become involved with one single factor and ignore the others? Physicians and scientists who are not afraid to think beyond convention need to address these problems.

CANCER

I T HAS BEEN SAID that more people live off cancer than ever die of it. If you total the money spent in the process of diagnosing and treating cancer, not to mention all the money spent doing research, it would rival the national debt. Cancer is big business, make no mistake. If we suddenly found the cause and a universal, inexpensive cure, it would probably throw the world economy into recession.

If you listen to the ads and public service announcements on television and listen to doctors talk, you'll find they proclaim that a cure for cancer would save thousands of lives. It's as if certain people were destined to die of cancer and of no other cause. If only we could cure cancer, they would live forever. It ain't so. Everyone dies of something. If not cancer, it will be an auto accident, pneumonia, AIDS, a broken hip, or a bullet from a jealous spouse. When the speed limit on interstate highways was lowered to 55 miles an hour, there was a big drop in deaths due to auto accidents, but no lives were actually saved. If you look at the death statistics for those years, you'll see that the total death rate did not fall. People simply died of something else, and so statistics show a slight increase in other causes of death. I am not denying the importance of the disease cancer, nor am I proposing we cease looking for its causes and effective treatment. What I do propose is that we put the problem into perspective and stop the hysteria.

Most cancers are preventable with the knowledge at hand today. Over half of all cancers are directly related to the use of tobacco. Nobody holds a gun to a person's head and forces him to smoke or dip snuff. Everyone knows tobacco is dangerous; the new user knows it when she lights up for the first time or he takes his first chew. Smoking causes cancer and emphysema and contributes to heart disease, high blood pressure, and strokes. Among the types of cancer directly linked to tobacco use are cancers of the lung, lip, tongue, mouth, larynx, kidney, urinary bladder, and others. This is common knowledge, and any teenager or adult who claims to be ignorant of these facts is either incredibly stupid or has his head stuck in the sand. I find it a bit difficult to feel too sorry for the person who smoked three packs a day for twenty years and then developed cancer of the lung. This is one thing I'm trying to get across with this book, that *people must take responsibility for their lives and accept the consequences of their actions without a lot of crying and sniveling.*

If I made a practice of walking around the roof edges of tall buildings, you would figure I was either crazy or had a death wish. When I fell, and we both know eventually I would, everyone would say I was asking for it and it served me right. I seriously doubt I would get much sympathy. So what's the difference whether I walk around roof edges or smoke? In both cases, I am performing an act, under my own free will, with full knowledge of the possible consequences. So much for that.

Cancer is caused by lack of communication at the intracellular level. I have no doubt this will someday be proven. Until then, it remains my own personal theory.

It is known that one can take epithelial cells from the intestinal lining of a tadpole and grow them in a tissue culture. Little bunches of cells can be grown fairly easily. As the cells grow and

Cancer

reproduce they form sheets of normal epithelial cells just as if they were still in the tadpole's intestine.

However, if one carefully teases the cells apart, separating them one from another so that the end result is *isolated* cells, something different happens. These single cells start to dedifferentiate. In other words, they change, losing the appearance and configuration of epithelial cells. They revert to a very primitive cell, not unlike a fertilized frog egg. As they grow and multiply, lo and behold, they produce a new tadpole. Wow, talk about exciting stuff!

When this same process is repeated using isolated epithelial cells from *older* tadpoles or frogs, it doesn't work so well. The cells, having been differentiated into epithelial cells for a longer time, find it harder to revert completely and attain their goal of behaving like a fertilized egg. They get partway back and appear to lose their direction. They become stuck. They reach a primitive state, to a large degree, but still retain some of the appearance of an epithelial cell. As they grow and multiply, they produce a wild mass of primitive cells dividing rapidly with no order or purpose. They look and behave exactly like a cancer.

This whole process has also been traced using specialized cells taken from the vascular bundles of carrots. By obtaining single, isolated cells, new carrots can be grown. The process of reproducing a new individual from a differentiated cell taken from non-reproductive tissue is called cloning.

The reason cloning can take place is that every cell in the entire organism carries in its nucleus the identical genes of the original fertilized egg. Remember in biology class when you studied cell division? The chromosomes in the nucleus would line up. Each chromosome would duplicate itself and then divide down the middle, with each new cell ending up an exact duplicate of the original. This process of mitosis, or cell division, is common to all living cells, whether they are plants, single-celled organisms, or more complicated animals such as butterflies or humans. This is the reason that

117

every individual cell in your body carries the same identical genes as were present when the first cell was formed by the union of your father's sperm with your mother's ovum. Each and every cell contains the potential for reproducing the whole organism. It carries a cellular blueprint, a concept, of what the whole individual should look like. Furthermore, the genetic material that furnished the blueprint to construct your body is identical to genetic material contained in the sperm and ovum of the first man and woman. Their genes have been replicated for millions of years and through countless generations.

The big question is, what makes a cluster of epithelial cells growing in the tissue culture produce sheets of normal cells growing and reproducing in an orderly fashion, while young isolated cells clone, and older isolated cells produce the cancerlike growth? The answer hinges upon important qualities of all living cells.

First, every cell knows its place and its destiny within the totality of the being of which it is a part. As the organism develops, cells adopt certain specific functions and assume the physical structure (differentiation) to perform those functions. One cell, upon finding itself where bone is destined to be, differentiates into an osteoclast and starts making bone. Another cell, immediately adjacent, differentiates into muscle; another changes into a connective tissue cell. This can occur because, deep within the cellular memory, within the genes and every atom constituting the protoplasm of the cells, lies the original concept of the organization of the total being. The cells operate and function smoothly within "The Plan" as long as communication exists between them.

If communication between the cells is interrupted, for any reason, a cell thinks it is isolated. In a sense, the isolated cell looks around, shrugs its shoulders at the task ahead, and attempts to start over. The genetic material is all there to produce another you. If it can just find its way back to its original form, the ovum, back through the process of dedifferentiation, then all will be well. The solitary cell, therefore, tries its best. But, like the cells from the older tadpoles, it only makes it partway. The cell divides and grows, making an imperfect mass of wildly multiplying cells. We call that confusion cancer.

For years, I read articles about cloning, and, for years, I discussed them with my father, a plant geneticist and morphologist. He had long before reasoned that cells were in themselves conscious, thought, had memory, and understood the concept of the whole organism. For the life of us, we could not figure out what might be the key to the process. What was involved in the intracellular communication system?

One night, at about four A.M., I was awakened from a sound sleep. I found myself sitting up in bed, fully awake, alert, my mind racing with excitement. I knew the answer! My friend Greg Satre calls such an event "a white light experience." The key to the communication system is Vitamin C.

It is known that Vitamin C plays a major role in allowing protein molecules to take part in biological processes. It acts as an electron acceptor. Unless protein can interact with other molecules, it is essentially "dead." To interact, a protein molecule has to get rid of an electron. Vitamin C accepts electrons from protein molecules, allowing them to be biologically active. Vitamin C is also an integral part of the electrical energy field, serving as the so-called intracellular cementing substance, binding cells together. For example, without adequate Vitamin C, scars and healed surgical incisions literally fall apart.

Exactly how the communication system works was not given to me, only that ascorbic acid is the key and loss of communication is the basic cause of malignancy. Viruses and carcinogenic agents such as tobacco tar play a role. Perhaps they, in some way, interfere with the function of Vitamin C. Whatever the details, I was informed during the "white light" event that if everyone took 8,000 to 10,000 milligrams of Vitamin C every day, cancer would be a rare disease. This would be a worthy experiment to try on a large scale. It would cost little, and no one would be harmed in the least.

Linus Pauling, along with Ewan Cameron, published a book on the effects of Vitamin C in treating advanced cancers. As one might expect, some cancers responded better than others. Some literally disappeared as long as the patient continued to take large amounts of the vitamin. My guess is that with enough C bathing the cancer cells, communication is restored, thereby affecting the growth and activity of the malignant cells. Whatever the reason, by taking huge amounts of Vitamin C, many of the cancers regress or disappear. Much research needs to be done in this area. The trouble is that once vitamins are mentioned, doctors and scientists are immediately prejudiced and turn a deaf ear.

There are other nutritional studies showing that the absence of other nutrients—such as Vitamin A (beta-carotene), Vitamin E, and roughage—also plays a role in allowing certain cancers to develop. All essential nutrients work in concert for the maintenance of body repair, growth, and health. For this reason, to concentrate on one single vitamin to the exclusion of other nutrients is to have a distorted view of the symphony of effects present when all essential nutrients are present.

In addition to the biochemical aspects of cellular changes we call cancer, there are psychological effects as well. As with every other disease, cancers can be initiated or allowed to grow if certain instructions are received from the subconscious mind. The potential for the development of malignancies is common within the body. As has already been stated, if the individual believes that she will develop a cancer, her cellular consciousness will not oppose or defend against the new growth. The body defends itself from tumors in much the same way it defends against infections. It is also possible for the subconscious mind, acting upon deeply implanted core beliefs, to instruct the cellular consciousness to dedifferentiate and develop a cancer. The cells do not perceive this action as being any other than totally cooperative, for they trust the information and instructions given to them by the subconscious mind. Any one or all factors may be operating within any given individual.

Cancer could largely be eliminated with good nutrition and attention to good health habits, along with a mature, balanced attitude toward life and a desire to remain healthy. Again, we humans create our environment and find that which we truly seek.

KINESIOLOGY AND CHIROPRACTIC

I MET A CHIROPRACTOR for the first time in the person of George Goodheart when I attended a weekend course on nutrition, biofeedback, and kinesiology where he was one of three individuals presenting the course. I was not actually interested in the kinesiology. I had gone to learn about biofeedback. Much to my surprise, I heard more information concerning anatomy, physiology, and pathology coming from the mouth of Dr. Goodheart than I had heard since graduating from medical school. George Goodheart, I came to discover, was a learned, brilliant physician and a superb teacher. I came away hooked on chiropractic, realizing that I had been guilty of an unwarranted, bigoted attitude toward chiropractors all my life.

There is no doubt that George Goodheart is a genius. My understanding of his contribution to chiropractic medicine may be inaccurate, since I'm not educated as a chiropractor. But it appears to me that he has firmly established chiropractic medicine as a truly scientific discipline. Examining a patient, identifying the cause of the problem, treating the patient, and then proving the treatment to be valid before the patient leaves the office is as scientific as one can get. Moreover, the treatment can be reproduced from patient to patient.

George admitted that what bothered him when he started practice and spurred him to find a better system than what he had learned in school was the inconsistency of the treatment results when the patients appeared to have the same problem. For example, a number of patients would present themselves with low-back pain. Their histories would be identical: They lifted something, were seized with pain in the back, and were unable to straighten up. On examination, they all appeared to have the same, identical problem. He would adjust them all the same way. One third would be fine and have no further problem. Another third would be fine only to return in a few days with the same symptoms and would require adjustment again and again. The final third he made worse! There had to be a reason.

Taking a multitude of different theories, concepts, and treatment procedures, Goodheart sorted them all out, determining what was effective and what did not work. He discovered the common underlying factors within these various disciplines and bound them into one integrated system of diagnosis and treatment. He borrowed the term "kinesiology," which is the science of anatomy as it applies to movement, and used it to embrace this new school of chiropractic medicine. Into this, he incorporated the concept of the physical body as an energy field. He and his followers probably understand the true nature of our physical being as a dynamic, shifting, multifaceted energy field as well as anyone in the world. They are able through various maneuvers to use the patient's body to "tell" the chiropractor what is wrong and what needs to be done. After the energy field is balanced, by whatever means, the doctor again uses the patient's body to confirm that what was done did indeed work. This is a scientific method, and no field of medicine does it any better.

Let me digress a moment and talk a bit about "science." To be accurate, we should speak of "scientific method" rather than science as a godlike entity having its own life. Science really implies knowledge gained through experimentation or practice. It is nothing more than a system of investigation where the conclusions are based upon observation of the results or effects of some thing or some action. That is not mysterious. The medical profession would lead you to believe that only their system is based on scientific principles and all other branches of health care are not.

In the chapter on maladaptive reactions, I explained how to use an arm muscle to determine food reactions and allergies. The same method is used to identify reflex points, as well as other areas of disease and injury that are present or not functioning in a proper manner. The doctor tests a muscle for strength and then has the patient touch a reflex point, for example. If the reflex center is malfunctioning, the test muscle becomes weak. It's all energy. It all works. It is unimportant that we do not know exactly why it works. Your medical doctor has no idea how the majority of drugs he prescribes work, so why is he complaining about the chiropractors?

At one time, I had in mind writing an article on the subject, on using this technique for identifying drug allergies. But I abandoned the project before I could write the paper, because my colleagues forbade me from doing any more kinesiology. The research project was a simple little double-blind experiment, the kind that doctors are trained to worship.

I decided to determine how accurate the muscle test was by applying it to patients with a penicillin allergy. I took three identical plastic pill containers, which were opaque so that it was impossible to see what they contained. Into one, I placed some penicillin capsules, and in the other two, I placed vitamin capsules. Every time a patient gave a history of penicillin allergy, I would test him with all three vials. If he tested weak with one vial, I would open it and identify the contents. I tested over fifty patients. In every instance, the test was accurate.

Occasionally, a patient would not become weak with any of the vials. On careful questioning it was obvious he was not allergic to penicillin. He had gotten the wrong impression or had been given the wrong diagnosis by the doctor. The accuracy of the test held up.

Chiropractors also incorporate elements of acupuncture into their treatment. In most states, they are not allowed to use needles, but touching the various acupuncture points is almost as effective in many cases. This technique is explained in Thie's book, *Touch for Health*. Incidentally, not allowing chiropractors to use needles is just another case of the medical profession's limiting of health-care alternatives.

For a period of about three and one-half years, I employed elements of chiropractic and kinesiology within my medical practice. It was very useful. One of my chiropractor friends, Bill Chapman, gave me a set of blocks and taught me to adjust a "category I" back strain. Combining this with a broad use of kinesiology, I had a lot of success with many of my patients.

One coal miner, Paul, was disabled. He had sustained a number of back injuries and had undergone a couple of back operations for a ruptured disc but was still unable to work. He experienced a lot of pain, most of the time. Our HMO would not pay for chiropractic treatment, but he wanted to try anyway. I referred him to a good chiropractor friend who was a skilled kinesiologist. He gave Paul a treatment that was effective and lasted for about three or four days. Then Paul's pain returned. He came to me, hardly able to walk, saying he was convinced the treatments would work but knew he could not afford to pay for the chiropractic treatments himself. I told him I would attempt to help.

Paul came in at the end of the day. I spent almost two hours working on him. As I recall, there were some twenty-four or -five different things I adjusted, including his category I back. He walked out of the office, pain free, and with his back in perfect alignment. Two days later he was in the same shape as before. I fixed him again. A couple of days later the same thing happened all over again. I called my chiropractor friend and asked him what was wrong. I was getting nowhere. He asked if as many things were still out of balance as there had been on the first treatment. I checked my notes and found that three or four of the abnormalities had not returned. He advised me to continue working, fixing what needed to be fixed, and, sooner or later, everything would remain adjusted.

He was right. It took two months of adjusting Paul, two or three times a week, before the adjustment wholly took. Paul was allowed to return to work after forfeiting his disability. He worked as a coal miner doing heavy work, shoveling on the belt line, for a little over a year. During that time, he remained pain free. Then he sustained a new back injury. By this time, the clinic had forbidden me to do any more chiropractic or kinesiology. Much as I wanted, there was no way I could treat him without their finding out. Several years later, when I resigned my position, Paul was again on disability, suffering constant, severe low-back pain.

In 1964, while on vacation, I slipped on some wet leaves while climbing around in Giant City State Park in southern Illinois. I fell, jamming one of my fingers as I landed in a heap on a ledge three feet below. My finger hurt so much that I was unaware I had also injured my back. An hour later, I drove several hundred miles home. Upon arriving, I could not get out of the car. I had to lift my legs with my hands and swing them to the ground. I waited for my back to get better. I took a few of Empirin with codeine for a while and suffered the pain but I never got well. I've always been able to absorb a lot of pain and just put it out of my mind.

Nineteen years later, my wife and I were planning a trip to China. I decided it was time to do something about my back, so I went to one of my chiropractor friends. He scolded me for not coming sooner and not having X-rays of my back. So I had some taken at the clinic. I had sustained a compression fracture of my third lumbar vertebra! My friend gave me a total of five treatments. On the first visit, he adjusted my skull and I left his office pain free. The next treatment was devoted to my feet, and I left pain free. I believe it was with the third treatment that he finally adjusted my back. As I said, he gave me a total of five adjustments, and I have been pain free ever since.

One problem is that kinesiology is not being taught in chiropractic schools. If it is, they have just started in the last few years. They, like the allopathic schools (medical schools that teach the use of drugs), are slow to accept and incorporate new concepts into their thinking and equally slow in eliminating that which does not work.

A bit of history is always interesting. Many years ago, I believe it was during the late 1930s or early 1940s, a counterfeit diploma mill was discovered to be operating in a big midwestern city. If memory serves me, an outfit in Kansas City was selling all sorts of professional diplomas. One could buy a chiropractic diploma for fifty dollars cash. The AMA made a big fuss, telling everybody who would listen what quacks chiropractors were. According to the AMA, and the impression given in the articles in the nation's newspapers, this was the way *all* chiropractors got their degrees. What a horrible bunch of people those low-down chiropractors were!

But today, we know that chiropractors are well-educated professionals. Chiropractic schooling is obviously different in many ways from the courses taught in allopathic schools. Their education is based upon the prevailing belief system adopted by their healing profession. If I had it to do over again, I would very likely go to chiropractic school, rather than be a medical physician. We need to remember that differences should not imply that one or the other belief is wrong.

Eventually, all healing professions will come to accept what chiropractors have already learned: that the physical body is an energy field, and distortions within the field account for the aberrations we refer to as illness. For healing to occur, the dynamic balance in the field must be restored, and often the ill or injured person may accomplish this all by himself. If he seeks the assistance of a healer, it matters very little whether the balance in the energy field is attained by the use of chemicals, herbs, adjustments, acupuncture, incantations, dances, or sand paintings. All are simply different ways of giving new instructions to the cells and enticing them to alter their functions and return to normal. In certain specific circumstances, some methods are more effective than others. This is to be expected. In some methods, it is possibly more important for the patient to be involved than in others, but for any of them to work effectively and permanently, the patient must believe in the validity of the treatment. Finally, some healers, regardless of their chosen methods, are just better than others. It is by the love of their patients and the force of their intent that they lead their patients to health.

Paul Tillich speaks of spiritual healing requiring three basic steps: reconciliation, faith, and surrender. These steps are also required in physical healing. First, there must be a balancing of the energy field, by whatever method of instruction to the cells involved. This is reconciliation. Second, the patient must have faith that she is healed, thereby altering her belief system and that of the bio-consciousness that says that she is sick. Third, she must be willing to surrender her illness, abandoning all the benefits attended by the illness.

No profession has a corner on wisdom, knowledge, or integrity. For every chiropractor who is incompetent, dangerous, and greedy, I can show you a medical doctor, dentist, or lawyer who is equally bad or worse. Attainment of an advanced educational degree does not ensure an individual has wisdom, knowledge, or integrity. All that is known is that he took specific classes and passed specific tests. We of the healing professions must band together, forget our differences, and accept one another as equal partners in the business of maintaining the health of our species. One of the best ways to accomplish this end is in the form of workshops where we can exchange knowledge, ideas, and goals. Then, last but not least, we all need to work together for the benefit of humankind.

TEMPORAL MANDIBULAR JOINT DYSFUNCTION

I N RECENT YEARS, there has been a lot of talk about temporal
mandibular joint dysfunction (TMJ disease). The definitive diagnosis and treatment of this problem belong in the territory of the dentists for two reasons. First, the medical profession doesn't understand it, knows little or nothing about it, at this point is unwilling to
learn, and mostly refuses to recognize it exists. Second, the treatment
can be properly performed only by a dentist knowledgeable in the
field of kinesiology. Temporal mandibular joint problems are serious
and cause untold thousands of people years of suffering and millions
of dollars every year in missed diagnoses and ineffective treatment.

If one examines the sensory portion of the brain lying along
a fold on the outside of the cerebral cortex, an interesting fact is evident. About seventy percent of the cells receive sensory input from
the mouth and its supporting structures, i.e., lips, teeth, tongue, muscles that move the jaw, and the joint where the jaw is hinged to the
skull. The remaining thirty percent is about equally divided between
the index finger and thumb together, and the rest of the body.

The relevance of this is that the oral cavity, the eating and
fighting apparatus, if you prefer, is extremely important to the well-
being of all animals. Eating means survival, and, since all our nour-

ishment is received through the mouth, it is of critical importance to be aware of every minute thing that goes wrong with the mouth. When the brain senses something is amiss, an alarm goes off. You are driven to have it fixed. If you don't believe it, the next time you get a bit of meat firmly wedged between your teeth, try to ignore it. Therefore, if the jawbone, or mandible, is not in ideal position and alignment, nerve endings located in the joint and muscles which support the mandible send messages to the brain, informing you that your jaw is not in the proper position to function as it should. This sense of location is called kinesthesia, the same as the sense of knowing the position of the various parts of the body without looking. We spoke of kinesthesia in the chapter on neurological development.

In response to this information that the jaw is out of ideal position, the brain relays directions to the muscles in an attempt to reposition the mandible so as to put the eating and fighting apparatus back in order. The result is often muscle spasm and pain. It is the whole set of symptoms brought about by an improper positioning or function of the temporal mandibular joint, for whatever reason, that sends patients to the doctor or dentist. The abnormal position of the mandible or abnormal action of the muscles is referred to as TMJ dysfunction. Problems with the TMJ are some of the most common causes of muscle tension headache. I knew of one case that lasted fourteen years, without letup, before the condition was diagnosed and treated.

What causes the TMJ to get out of alignment? The joint is one of the most complicated in the body and is subject to a lot of wear and tear. The stress ranges from grinding the teeth to trauma sustained in falls and fights. More common than trauma is loss of vertical dimension. This is the distance between the mandible and the maxillary bone located above it. The loss of vertical dimension may be caused by the loss of one or more teeth, which allows the others to shift and the bite to collapse, resulting in over-closure of the mouth. At other times, it is caused by ill-fitting dentures. More often than not, when a dentist is fitting a patient for dentures, he or she is not fully aware of the importance of restoring the proper vertical dimension and, likely, is uncertain how to determine the exact vertical dimension in any given patient. At other times, the patient may have gone without teeth so long that the muscles have contracted, making it impossible for the dentist to open the bite sufficiently with the first set of dentures. Most people are unwilling to go to the expense of having the dental restoration done properly.

So an alarm goes off: "My jaw is out of alignment, or closed so much I can't get it open wide enough to eat or fight!" Muscles go into spasm in an attempt to pull the mandible into its proper position, pain ensues, and the poor soul is off to the M.D. with a headache or earache. The same nerve supplies sensation to both the ear and the TMJ, so an earache is about as common a symptom as a headache. Frequently, the pain is severe and constant. It is not uncommon for the patients or their insurance companies to spend thousands upon thousands of dollars before the condition is diagnosed and someone qualified is found to treat it.

I made it a practice when seeing an adult with a headache or earache to check out the mouth and TMJ. About half the time, I would discover missing molars or ill-fitting dentures. Using a kinesiology maneuver, it was a simple thing to confirm the diagnosis. I'd test an arm muscle for strength the same way I would test for a food intolerance and then start placing tongue blades between the patient's teeth, opening the bite until maximum strength was achieved. One too many tongue blades and the muscle immediately became weak. It was not unusual for a thickness of four or five tongue blades to be required to reestablish the proper vertical dimension.

The hard part came in obtaining adequate definitive diagnosis and treatment for my patients. Daniel Alexander, a dentist in Bellaire, Ohio, happens to be one of my best friends and is an expert on TMJ problems. In fact, he taught me everything I know about the subject, and what he knows would fill a big book on the subject. The problem was that our HMO, like so many others, would not pay for the treatment. Only two or three other doctors in the clinic even recognized the condition existed, so I had no luck convincing our HMO to include this common problem on their list of covered services. Inclusion of TMJ treatment would have increased the monthly premium a couple of dollars, and the premiums were already quite high. Our clinic was in stiff competition with another HMO in the area, and, as long as it did not include TMJ in its list of covered services, we could not afford to, either. In most cases, private insurance would not pay for the treatment, either—although this has begun to change in the last few years. The reason private insurance companies have not included the condition into the formula when they calculate their premiums is financial as well. Then, too, probably nobody on their medical advisory staffs accept the condition as valid. It is a great dodge, the dentists saying it is a medical problem, and the doctors claiming it is dental. By keeping the controversy going on endlessly, neither have to face their responsibilities.

Dan and I worked closely together. I referred him a lot of patients, and he was successful with everyone he treated. I doubt he even charged a couple of the people who were in dire need of relief but could not pay. With others who could not afford the treatment, I at least had the satisfaction of knowing I had made the correct diagnosis and had not sent them on that endless merry-go-round of CT scans, neurologists, and psychiatrists, as most of my colleagues were prone to do.

To give a specific example, the wife of one of the doctors in the clinic had a severe TMJ syndrome, resulting in more or less constant severe headaches that had been present for years. At a social gathering one evening, she asked me to check her out, and, later, during the course of a complete physical, I confirmed that TMJ dysfunction was her problem. I suggested she see Dr. Alexander, since she already went to Dan for her dental care. Her husband, however, refused to accept TMJ dysfunction as the cause of her head pain. In fact, he refused to believe there *was* such a thing as TMJ dysfunction causing symptoms. He had not learned about it in medical school or in his internal medicine residency, so, of course, it could not exist. She was unwilling to go against her husband's opinion by insisting he allow Dan to treat her. So, she went without treatment. Last year, Dan told me she had finally come to him for treatment after all that time, a good ten years. He corrected her problem and relieved her headache. Her husband confessed he had been wrong all those years. At least he was honest enough to admit it, but his refusal to accept a new idea caused his wife years of needless suffering.

Treatment can be very involved, depending upon the original cause of the difficulty and the resulting problems that need to be corrected. New dentures and intraoral splints are often required, alone or in combination. In severe cases, surgery on the joint may be required. Occasionally, when one of my patients could not afford treatment, or as a temporary measure while awaiting an appointment with the dentist, I would tape some tongue blades together after determining the number required to restore the vertical dimension. Then, I'd have the patient gently hold them between his or her teeth at the onset of a headache or earache. I recall one lady with horrible headaches. Her dentures were so shallow that it took nine tongue blades to approximate normal alignment of her mandible. At the start of a headache, she would pop the bundle of tongue blades in her mouth and the headache would disappear within a few minutes and remain gone sometimes for days. With many patients, this crude splint was often effective—and it cost nothing.

Health insurance companies, both medical and dental, need universally to accept temporal mandibular joint dysfunction as a real, honest-to-God entity and include diagnosis and treatment into their coverage. The medical profession needs to start making the diagnosis where it is appropriate and referring these cases to the dentists so they can apply their knowledge in confirming the diagnosis and treating the condition. And both professions need to quit the game of "It's your problem. No it ain't, it's yours."

Then, the burden will fall directly on the dental profession. Only that profession is potentially equipped to diagnose and treat the condition properly, but, at present, not enough dentists are adequately trained to do so. Often, it is poor dentistry that is the cause of the problem in the first place. Someone needs to pick up the ball and help the patients. When professions disagree, the patient always pays.

T E N

REACTIVE
HYPOGLYCEMIA

L OW BLOOD SUGAR is referred to in a rather mystical fashion
by many people and a lot of doctors. Some physicians flatly
refuse to recognize the condition while others don't appear to
understand it at all. It will be helpful if you have some basic
understanding of how the body controls the amount of glucose circulating in the blood at any one time.

Sugars and starches are digested and absorbed from the
intestinal tract as glucose, which is carried directly to the liver
through a huge network of veins called the portal system. In the liver,
much of the glucose is converted to a compound called glycogen,
which is stored in the liver as a reserve to be reconverted to glucose in
emergencies. The rest is allowed to enter the general circulation,
passing directly to the heart, where it is pumped throughout the body
for use in the metabolism of every cell. In muscle, some is converted
to glycogen and stored there, just as it is stored in the liver.

As the sugar level of the blood rises following a meal, special
cells within the pancreas are triggered to produce insulin. The
insulin, released into the bloodstream, attaches to the cell walls of
the tissues, opening the door, in a manner of speaking, for the glucose to enter the cells. Glucose is used by every cell in the body to

supply energy for life and to perform whatever task the particular cell is designed to accomplish.

The total amount of glucose normally circulating in the bloodstream amounts to about two teaspoonfuls. Certain physiologic mechanisms are constantly at work to maintain the blood sugar level in a dynamic balance of supply and demand. Exercise lowers the sugar level as skeletal muscle burns glucose to do its work. Insulin, in response to the rise in glucose, is produced in a greater amount causing the cells of the body to take up glucose, thereby lowering the level found in the bloodstream.

On the opposite side of the balance, glucagon, produced in the pancreas, converts glycogen back to glucose, raising the sugar level. ACTH is a hormone produced by the adrenal cortex. You learned about it in relation to stress (*see* page 60). It also raises blood sugar levels by converting protein and fat in the body to glucose. During times of starvation and severe chronic stress, this effect of ACTH can be quite pronounced. The stress encountered in a rapid drop in blood sugar also triggers a release of adrenaline from the adrenal glands. Adrenaline raises the blood sugar as well and, at the same time, is responsible for many of the symptoms associated with a low blood sugar.

The mechanisms described in this rough sketch of blood-sugar dynamics are responsible for maintaining the glucose level within a narrow normal range, even during times of fasting and starvation. Unless you have some problem with your physiology, you do not develop a low blood sugar before breakfast or by skipping a couple of meals.

If one has a tumor involving the islet cells, it usually makes insulin. The excessive insulin will cause true attacks of low blood sugar, even when you're eating normally. This is a very rare condition, so don't start imagining you have one. In forty-four years of practice, I had only one case, and I spent a lot of time and ran a lot of tests looking for another. They are dramatic, interesting cases, and a lot of fun to work up and prove. They just aren't to be found, except in rare instances.

Juvenile diabetics are true diabetics, suffering a condition caused by an inadequate amount of insulin being produced by the islet cells in the pancreas. To survive, they must regulate their intake of food and inject insulin in various forms into their bodies.

But adult onset diabetes, as you learned in Chapter 3, is not due to the lack of insulin, but to a maladaptive reaction to some food. The disease should be given another name. Insulin levels in these folks are actually *higher* than in healthy people. The pancreas puts out more and more insulin in response to the elevated sugars, but it just doesn't work very well. The stress reaction takes one of two forms. It may affect the insulin receptors on the surface of the cells, rendering them unable to accept the insulin. Another possibility is that it affects the insulin directly, altering that part of the molecule which attaches to the receptors. But whatever the reason, the insulin doesn't work.

Reactive hypoglycemia, or low blood sugar, is not a strange or rare disorder. During my practice I ran perhaps 200 or 300 six-hour glucose tolerance tests on various patients. I came to the conclusion that reactive hypoglycemia is an extremely common, *normal* response to the act of consuming a large amount of sugar in a short time. The condition is called "reactive" because it is a reaction to eating sugar (in contrast to other pathologic conditions where the sugar may become low as a result of some disease process or a quirk in the body physiology). Reactive hypoglycemia occurs simply because the body physiology is not designed to handle huge amounts of sugar suddenly dumped into the system. It's that simple.

When our prehistoric ancestors were in the process of evolving their physiology millions of years ago, they did not regularly eat large amounts of sugar. For this reason, the human body does not have the machinery to handle raw sugar without some problem. Except for occasional feasts of honey, ancient humans' carbohydrates came in the form of fruit, roots, and grass seed, and many of those foods were seasonal. Of course, the food stuffs had to be digested, so the sugar entered the system over a period of several hours.

When you have pancakes and syrup for breakfast, one ounce of syrup contains seventy-five grams of sugar, which is the amount of sugar in six apples, and that doesn't even count the starch in the pancakes themselves. If you are like me, you like a lot of syrup; I'm more apt to eat a couple of ounces. That's twelve apples! In the first place, if you could eat twelve apples at once, it would take you a lot longer than it takes you to eat breakfast. In the second place, the sugar in the apple has to be digested, so it is not absorbed as rapidly as the syrup.

The sugar in the syrup hits your body like a ton of bricks. Within five or ten minutes, *at the most,* the sugar is absorbed from your intestine, overwhelming the liver in its attempt to store it all. The glucose surges into the bloodstream, triggering the islet cells into action. This is an *abnormal* situation, and the islet cells wave their arms and become hysterical, producing a lot of insulin, much more than they should. After all, this is not just a normal day for them. This is panic time. With all that insulin, the blood sugar drops like a rock, diving to levels below normal. This rapid drop in blood sugar triggers off a release of adrenaline which produces the same set of symptoms as are experienced by a diabetic when he takes too much insulin or does not eat. Most people become sweaty, weak, faint, their hearts pound, they may feel numb and tingly. If the blood sugar drops low enough, the brain cells and nerves cannot function, and the person may become depressed or unconscious or appear drunk.

Given time, the body calls upon its reserves of glycogen, the blood sugar rises, and everything returns to normal. Keep in mind this is a physiological reaction, so no danger is present, as there is when a massive dose of insulin is taken by mistake, which sometimes happens with diabetics. The insulin used in treating diabetes is often altered to produce a sustained effect, so a hypoglycemic reaction produced by these altered insulins may continue for hours if the person does not receive help in the form of candy or intravenous glucose. Reactive hypoglycemia will not cause anything terrible to happen unless you become dizzy and hurt yourself.

What confuses a lot of doctors is that not everyone develops symptoms during bouts of low blood sugar. Others develop symptoms when the sugar level has apparently remained in normal ranges. These things lead many physicians to deny the existence of the condition. Let me explain. First of all, no two people are alike. If you took a large group of people, lined them up and hit each one of them equally hard on the shin with a sledgehammer, some would get a broken leg, others would sustain a bruise, and a few would say "ouch." Nor does everyone exhibit the same symptoms when his blood sugar falls. Doctors like to think that people react the same in all situations. Intellectually, they know it is not true, but when dealing with patients, they tend to go on that premise. Look at the doses of medicine given. They are careful to calculate the dose of medicine for a child, but when it comes to adults, a ninety-pound woman is apt to get the same amount of medicine as a 300-pound man.

To understand why an individual will have symptoms when the sugar remains at fairly normal values, it helps to know what a normal three-hour glucose tolerance curve looks like. The figure below shows a normal curve. The shaded strip across the graph indi-

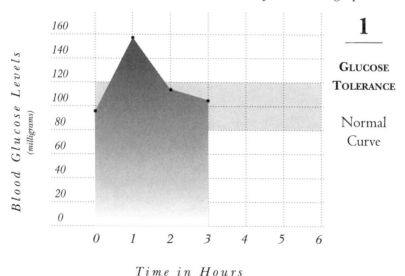

1

GLUCOSE TOLERANCE

Normal Curve

Blood Glucose Levels
(milligrams)

Time in Hours

cates the normal range of blood sugar during a fasting state or a couple of hours after a regular meal. This varies between 80 and 120 milligrams of glucose in 100 cubic centimeters (about three ounces) of blood. An hour after drinking a dose of glucose, the level will rise, but not above about 160. At the end of the second hour it should be back into the normal range again. If it goes too high or does not fall back to normal range quickly enough, the person is considered to be a diabetic.

The problem is that 100 grams of glucose, which is the standard amount given during a test, is a *huge* slug of sugar—far more than the body is designed to handle. If the tolerance test is continued for another three hours, lots of interesting things can be observed. The curve will almost always look something like this:

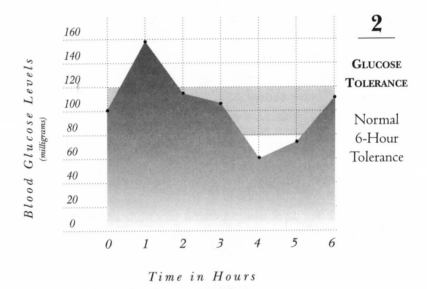

2

GLUCOSE TOLERANCE

Normal 6-Hour Tolerance

Time in Hours

Usually during the fourth hour, the patient will show symptoms of low blood sugar. On this particular curve, the blood sugar appears to have dropped to about 60, and that is not low enough to trigger a reaction. This happened to be the graph of one of my patients who became very ill between the third and fourth hour, sweating, shaking, numb, and almost passing out. The reason for the seeming discrepancy was that the sugars were drawn at hourly intervals. A lot of things can happen in an hour. I was anxious to document what I knew had occurred, so I could attempt to educate some of my colleagues. I talked the patient into letting me repeat the test a few days later when her arm got over being sore. She was on a prepaid program, so there was no expense for her.

On the repeat test, I had the laboratory draw blood every fifteen minutes throughout the fourth hour. This is how her glucose curve looked:

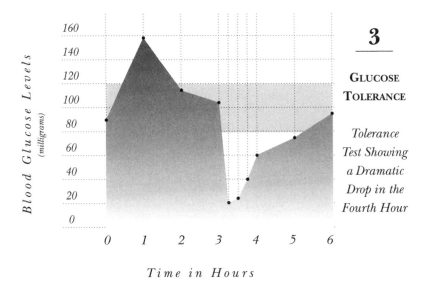

3
———
GLUCOSE TOLERANCE

Tolerance Test Showing a Dramatic Drop in the Fourth Hour

Time in Hours

Obviously, she had one hell of a drop fifteen minutes into the fourth hour. Her blood sugar had started to recover by the fifth hour and continued to rise until it finally attained normal levels in the sixth hour. It was the bad luck of the timing. One could say the luck of the draw. If the drop to 20 had occurred fifteen minutes earlier, it would have shown on the first test. No doctor would have argued the case. My colleagues were polite when I showed them the lady's sugar curves, but I could not see where it changed their general attitude toward the subject of low blood sugar.

One other point: Symptoms seem to be triggered more by the rapidity in which the sugar level falls than the absolute level itself. When treating an out of control diabetic, we sometimes observe symptoms if the sugar drops rapidly from, say, 400 to 120. One hundred twenty is within normal physiologic range.

Hypoglycemic reactions are so common when doing six-hour tolerance tests that I all but gave up doing them. If a patient reported symptoms after eating sweets, there was no point in putting her through the time, expense, and pain of being stuck seven or eight times just to have some numbers to look at. To run a test on a patient with a solid history of hypoglycemic reactions makes about as much sense as going out into a January blizzard with a thermometer to document that it's cold outside. It matters little whether it is zero or five below. It is the same with low blood sugar. Whether the sugar falls to 50 or 30 is of no clinical importance.

There were situations when the circumstances were not clear. I had one man come to see me complaining there were times he walked into door edges and bumped into tables and chairs. He claimed he could not see them. The problem was inconsistent. Sometimes he had trouble and sometimes not. I did a complete examination and could find nothing. He appeared to be a perfectly healthy young man; however, one does not ignore symptoms of that nature. I ordered a battery of lab tests and referred him to the optometrist to have his visual fields plotted. I wanted to see if there was some defect in the optic nerve that might account for his loss of peripheral vision. What I had in mind was a brain tumor.

The morning he saw the optometrist, he had also gone to the lab for the blood tests. On a hunch, I had included a six-hour glucose tolerance test along with the others. The glucose tolerance started at 8:00 and the optometrist plotted his fields at about 10:00.

He came hurrying over to my office saying the patient had some constriction of his fields and informed me he wanted to do them again, as soon as he saw his next patient. It was about 11:30 when he plotted the fields for the second time and found them to be far worse. The patient had now lost all his peripheral vision. All he could see was directly in front of him. The optometrist thought he had gone nuts. Visual fields don't change that rapidly. He informed me what he had found the second time around and explained he was having the man return later in the afternoon when he was not so rushed with patients. At that hour, he could take more time and have the other optometrist double-check him. At 4:00, the fields were perfectly normal. The poor optometrist was totally confused.

Dumb me; I had actually forgotten I had ordered the glucose tolerance. When the laboratory report was delivered to me the next morning all the answers fell into place. At 10:00, when the first fields were done, he was two hours into the glucose tolerance. He was starting to develop a severe low blood sugar reaction. The blood sugar was down to 60. By 11:30, when his fields were plotted for the second time, the blood sugar had fallen to 35 and he had lost all this peripheral vision. No wonder the poor guy ran into the furniture. During the late afternoon, the blood sugar had recovered to normal as had his vision.

When the patient returned for his laboratory reports I questioned him again concerning other symptoms he might have neglected to mention. Loss of peripheral vision was his only apparent symptom. As I stated earlier, brain and nerve cells are extremely sensitive to low levels of sugar and do not function normally under those conditions. That accounted for the dysfunction of his optic nerves. If he had not had the glucose tolerance run at the same time he was having his fields plotted, the cause of his problem might not have been discovered—at least not for a long time. I shudder to think of all the scans, tests, and consultations he would have been put through. I wonder what sort of repressed sexual problem the psychiatrist would have presumed him to have.

Self-diagnosis of low blood sugar episodes is rather simple and highly accurate. All that is required is a moderate amount of attention to how you feel and what you have eaten. The symptoms fall into two groups: those that are caused by the release of adrenaline and those due to changes in the function of the nervous system and brain. It is unnecessary to try distinguishing between the two. The release of adrenaline results in a feeling of mild anxiety, sweating, pounding heart, trembling, slight dizziness, and sometimes hunger or nausea. The changes in brain function can result in many of the same symptoms: dizziness, confusion, visual disturbances, depression or anxiety, difficulty speaking, loss of hearing, and even loss of consciousness. As frightening as these may sound, the symptoms are self-limiting if you do nothing but wait.

Usually, symptoms come on between two and three hours after eating something sweet, such as a soft drink or candy. If it is eaten on an empty stomach, the sugar gets into your system more rapidly than if the same amount of sugar were taken during the course of a meal. Sweet breakfasts often contain little other food, so symptoms between 10:00 and 11:00 in the morning are common. Some individuals are more sensitive than others, and even if they have a heavy meal and follow it with a sweet dessert they may develop symptoms. If you develop some of the symptoms I have mentioned, think back to what you ate two or three hours before. The chances are that you consumed a lot of sugar. If you are uncertain, one good way is to take a day when you can afford to have trouble and eat nothing but a very sweet meal such as pancakes with loads of syrup, coffee loaded with sugar or a soft drink. Then sit back and observe how you feel for the next few hours. You can then decide what course of action to take.

The cure is simple. If sweets make you shaky, sweaty, and feel funny—don't eat sweets. Like the old joke: "Doctor, it only hurts when I laugh." "Don't laugh." When you develop symptoms, the worst thing you can do is to eat candy, drink a soft drink, or have a doughnut and coffee. That only triggers a second rise of blood sugar with another precipitous drop and more trouble. The answer is—don't laugh; I mean don't eat sweets. If the symptoms are such that you cannot hold out long enough for your body to correct the problem, then eating an apple or orange is OK.

For most people, going overboard with a rigid sugar-free diet, eating snacks between meals, and such is overkill. Keep it simple. Just avoid obviously sweet things like desserts, pop, and candy. Once in a while, if you want, and the symptoms are not all that uncomfortable, for heaven's sake have some pancakes and syrup. Ignore the symptoms and wait until lunch. By noon, the symptoms should be gone in any case.

Above all, reactive hypoglycemia is not a disease—it is a normal response to taking in a large amount of simple sugar in a short period of time. It is not mysterious, except in the minds of many doctors and patients who are poorly informed. I heard some poor soul on a talk show recently telling of the years and money spent before having the condition diagnosed. She claimed she had had numerous three-hour glucose tolerance tests and seen several physicians before she had a six-hour test performed. Then, it apparently had been misread. The interesting thing was that the woman had a good idea concerning her diagnosis. Still, she persisted in running from doctor to doctor to find one who would confirm the diagnosis and run a six-hour test. Most folks can make the diagnosis for themselves. The average person gives himself a glucose tolerance test at breakfast every morning and flunks it by noon.

People have to quit expecting others to do their thinking for them. This not only applies to your health, but to politics, birth control, abortion, economics, everything. That's why God gave everyone a brain, not just a select few. Someone once said that the beginning of civilization occurs when people start letting others do their thinking. It may well be true, and, if so, we need to rethink the way we live.

HYPNOSIS

H YPNOSIS has already been mentioned a number of times throughout the book. It is such a useful and powerful tool that the subject deserves its own chapter. Unfortunately, few doctors know anything about it, much less how to use it in their practices.

In Western culture, hypnosis was first reported by Mesmer, a Austrian physician. It became known as Mesmerism and gave rise to the verb "to mesmerize," which, of course, means to cast a spell on someone. Like so many things, it had been known and used in Eastern cultures for at least 2,000 years before it reached us. (In line with European-American thinking, a concept or practice doesn't count unless discovered by someone of the white race and written into a scientific article.)

Anyway, Mesmer was claiming rather fantastic medical cures using his discovery. He had so many patients that he could not see them all individually, so he "passed his power" into a tub of water. He placed a number of metal rods into the tub and patients would simply hold onto the rods. That way, he could treat as many people at one time as he had rods or could crowd around the tub. The patients reported marvelous results. He caused such a stir in Europe that word spread to the United States. George Washington, who was then president, sent Benjamin Franklin to France to investigate what was going on. Franklin returned saying Mesmerism didn't appear to be anything other than suggestion. Score a big A+ for Ben Franklin.

Classical hypnosis is an altered state of consciousness in which the mind concentrates exclusively on specific suggestions given to it. The suggestions can come from the hypnotist or from the subject. In addition, during this altered state the analytical portion of the conscious mind—that part that says white is white and sharp things hurt—appears to be temporarily circumvented. Suggestions given during a hypnotic state seem to bypass the conscious mind and go directly to the subconscious. This allows the subconscious mind to act freely, uninhibited by the conscious mind and the ego. Hypnosis imparts no special abilities to the individual. Anything that can be accomplished in a hypnotic state can be done in the unhypnotized state. Hypnosis only facilitates the process by bypassing our fears and doubts and the objections of the conscious mind.

Hypnosis makes it possible to recall events and experiences long forgotten. Freud knew this, and all his early work was done with his patients hypnotized. Somewhere along the line, peer pressure must have gotten to him, for he abandoned hypnosis in favor of free association. Had Freud continued with hypnosis, I seriously doubt he would have persisted in his theory that almost every problem besetting humankind is based on repressed sexual frustrations as he himself suffered. He would have come to realize that the subconscious mind is to be trusted and not to be viewed as a hidden, subterranean level of awareness, bending lives into horrid, sick adventures. In any case, hypnosis is an extremely useful and accurate method of recalling forgotten events in this—and perhaps other—lives.

I became involved with hypnosis in the mid-1950s, when I took a course from a man named Dave Elman. I owe a lot to him. It was through hypnosis that I learned much about the effect that the mind has on the body. Dave Elman was an old stage hypnotist, like his father before him. He had given up his entertainment career and was traveling the country teaching hypnosis to physicians and dentists. He would target six or seven cities in an area and drive from town to town teaching a lesson in each. Then he would return to the first city and teach lesson number two, and so on. About ten or so of us in the Champaign area enrolled in his class. It included, besides myself, a couple of obstetricians, a podiatrist, a couple of dentists, and several other general practitioners. Our class was on Sunday night; during the week, we would practice what we had been taught in the foregoing classes.

Dave Elman was a fantastic clinical hypnotist, and what he may not have known about the theory of hypnosis he more than made up for with his experience and practical knowledge. One evening, I took a friend to class with me. He was a professor of psychology and skilled in hypnosis. After class, I asked my friend what he thought of the course. He said, "That old man doesn't know the first thing about the modern theories of hypnosis, but he is the best clinical hypnotist I have ever seen in my life. Learn everything you can from him." He went on to say, "But, what do we really know about hypnosis? Maybe he is right and all our modern theories are wrong. Who knows, and who cares?"

I took to it like the proverbial duck to water and began using it in my practice. I used it in obstetrics and delivered quite a number of babies using hypno-anesthesia. I performed numerous minor surgical procedures using the technique for anesthesia. I used it to help people stop smoking and to break habits, and I did a fair amount of psychotherapy using hypnosis as a vehicle for recall. Through the use of hypnosis, I began to appreciate the power of the mind to affect physical events occurring within the body. It was in Dave Elman's classes that I learned how to dispel conditioned reflexes and cure a lot of physical ills. At the time, I did not know anything about cellular consciousness and did not fully comprehend the reasons behind the excellent results I enjoyed. That knowledge came much later in my career.

To illustrate the value and lasting effectiveness of hypnosis and posthypnotic suggestions, let me relate a case in which I supplied the anesthesia via posthypnotic suggestion for a woman having her baby in Hawaii.

During the summer term at the university, I saw a young lady pregnant with her first baby. Her husband was in graduate school, and they were in Illinois only for the one term. Then they returned to Hawaii. She came to me for prenatal care on three occasions. During her first visit, she expressed an interest in hypnosis, so I hypnotized her and gave her a number of suggestions relating to her pregnancy and delivery. The lady said she wanted to have her baby using hypnosis for anesthesia but felt certain there would be no doctor in Hawaii who would hypnotize her. She was such an excellent subject, I told her she could do it by herself if she wanted. I hypnotized her three times on each of the prenatal visits she made that summer.

The suggestions were that when the contractions began, she would start to relax. She would feel the contractions as a pleasant pressure, and she would look forward to the next, for each one meant she was that much closer to seeing her baby. I suggested that as the contractions became stronger she would become even more comfortable.

I assumed the doctors and nurses would be talking about pain and hurting, so I suggested that at the mere hint by anyone that she was in pain or uncomfortable in any way, she would become even more comfortable and think the remark amusing if not outright funny. I went on to suggest that as the baby's head began to press on the pelvic floor and began to emerge, her entire pelvic area would become as numb as if she had been given a spinal anesthetic.

On each occasion that I hypnotized her, I had her practice making various parts of her body numb and then had her stick hypodermic needles into the anesthetized area to further enforce the effectiveness of the hypnosis.

She and her husband returned to Hawaii. Several months later, after she delivered her eight and one-half pound girl, she wrote to me. The posthypnotic suggestions had been entirely successful. The doctors and nurses would enter the labor room saying, "You've got to be having pain." She would laugh and giggle, saying she was fine and felt great. When it came time to deliver the baby, the doctor told her he was going to do an episiotomy and insisted upon doing a pudendal block. She said she was so numb she could not even feel his fingers when he examined her. But she consented to the block in order to humor the nice, confused doctor.

This was successful for two reasons. First, the patient was highly motivated, wanting above all for the hypnosis to be effective. Second, the girl was a superb subject, and I prepared her well, anticipating the negative suggestions I knew would surround her, turning them around for her advantage.

What turned out to be my most exciting discovery was that people could feel the workings of their bodies under hypnosis. They could feel their hearts beat, not just the thump, but actually the blood spurting into the aorta and the pulse of the arteries as the blood flowed throughout the body. They could perceive the contraction of their stomachs and intestines, urine running down the ureters into their bladders, and their gallbladders contract. Wow, it was exciting!

In an effort to validate this information, I hypnotized patients with undiagnosed illnesses or symptoms. I would then investigate their organs one at a time and have the patient pinpoint the source of the difficulty. After the hypnosis, I would obtain tests and X-rays, and, sure enough, the patients were invariably right. Subconsciously, every patient knew what was wrong with his or her body, whether it was an ulcer, gallstones, or whatever. The bio-consciousness of the body cannot be fooled, and even though we are unaware of it, it is in constant communication with the subconscious mind.

Using hypnosis, I observed the power of the mind on the body physiology and the actions and behavior of the cells. These effects were often visible in a very dramatic fashion. I hypnotized one lady and asked her if she would allow me to burn her forearm if I promised she would feel no pain and the burn would heal quickly without a scar. She agreed, a bit reluctantly, but she agreed. I placed her into a trance, suggested that her forearm was numb and then pressed the end of a wooden letter opener that was on my desk against the skin of her forearm. As I pressed the opener on her arm I told her she would not feel it burning. After about a minute I removed the letter opener and, before my eyes, the skin that had been beneath the opener became red and swollen and a blister formed. Reinforcing the suggestion she would have no pain and the burn would heal within an hour, I brought her out of trance. Then I explained what I had done. Before she left the office, the "burn" had begun to disappear. If the subconscious mind can produce a burn and a blister, then it can produce other alterations in the body physiology and either create diseases or heal diseases, according to the body-mind commitment. What we believe will happen, happens.

One of my patients was a professor of psychology whose area of research at one time had been hypnosis. He was the friend I had taken to one of Dave Elman's classes. We frequently discussed the subject of hypnosis and shared what we had learned and what could be accomplished using it. One Sunday morning, he called saying he was having some pain and soreness in his belly and needed a house call. Barry was a good-sized man. In fact, he was fat, but he was also built like a brick outhouse with a powerful body and heavily muscled arms and legs. I tried to examine him, but, with all the muscle and about five inches of fat, there was no way to be certain what I was feeling. He suggested I do one of my "organ interviews." I had hypnotized Barry on several occasions and we had a cue arranged, so I scratched the left side of my head and Barry went into a trance.

I suggested his subconscious mind allow him to perceive the feelings from the muscles of his right forearm. He described a peculiar quivering in the muscles which other hypnosis subjects had reported. He suggested that the quivering he was perceiving was muscle tonus, and I agreed with him. Then I told him to feel his stomach, suggesting that since he had not had breakfast, he probably would feel very little.

"No, it's full of food," he replied. "It's just laying there. It must be what I ate last night. It hasn't emptied at all."

Then I suggested he feel his appendix. Barry reported he felt nothing whatever. I thought, "Come on, Bonnett, that's asking too much," so I enlarged the area, suggesting he feel the last foot or two of his small bowel, the appendix, and the first foot of his colon. Immediately, he winced, saying that was where the trouble lay.

In the hospital, his white count was over 20,000, confirming he had some sort of inflammatory process going on, probably appendicitis. Barry told me he had read some reports that people continued to hear even while under a general anesthetic, and he asked that I be sure to say something while he was asleep which he would likely remember. Afterward, we could hypnotize him and see if he could recall the remark.

Being Sunday, the only person I could find to assist in surgery was an OB man who referred all his general surgery to me. Barry was anesthetized, and George and I had finished scrubbing and were being gowned when the obstetrical floor called saying one of his patients had just arrived, in the process of delivering. I told George to take care of his delivery and return; meanwhile I would open the belly with the capable assistance of the scrub nurse.

Barry, as I have said, was fat, and the anesthetist had a terrible time getting him deep enough to be adequately relaxed. Adipose tissue tends to soak up anesthetic like a sponge. First, he vomited about a quart of undigested food. He'd been right about his stomach being full. With poor relaxation of the abdominal wall, I had considerable trouble exposing his appendix. Finally, after a struggle, I was able to get to the appendix and found it extremely short and stubby, about the size of the end of my thumb. It was acutely inflamed. I had some difficulty getting it clamped off, removed, and the stump inverted. Just as I was finishing, George returned.

By this time Barry had enough anesthetic in him so he was nicely relaxed, and I had a good view of the area. George pulled the end of the cecum up into the incision so I could make certain there were no small bleeders I had not tied. Lo and behold, there was his appendix, hiding behind his cecum. What I had found and removed was an infected diverticulum of the cecum. It had formed exactly where the appendix was normally located, or at least it appeared to be. A diverticulum is a small finger-like pouch protruding from within the bowel out through the wall of the gut.

"Well, Barry," I said in a loud voice. "Here you are trying to pass yourself off as a fat Jew and there's nothing kosher about you at all. You didn't have appendicitis, you had a cecal diverticulitis." I explained all was OK, and we were going to take out his normal appendix as well.

Barry was told nothing of what happened in the operating room. The next day I hypnotized him and suggested he go back in time to when he was put to sleep. These were his words.

"I can hear you talking with the nurse and the other doctor.—My god, George is going to leave! You're going to operate alone? I guess it's all right or you wouldn't be doing it.—I missed that; there was some noise around my ears from the anesthetic mask.—I can hear you talking with the nurse. —(laughing) You son-of-a-bitch, what do you mean I'm not kosher, but what the hell is a cecal diverticulum?" Out of hypnosis, we enjoyed a good laugh. The experiment had worked. People do hear what is said while they are asleep with a general anesthetic. It is just that they ordinarily cannot remember without the aid of hypnosis.

The next day, Barry had a superficial wound infection. Fat tissue has poor resistance to infection and Barry had about five inches of fat between the skin and the abdominal wall. In spite of my using a drain, he had a big superficial wound abscess. As I was taking out a couple of skin stitches to facilitate drainage, Barry suggested I hypnotize him and tell his body how to get rid of the infection. He had read other articles from Russia in which visualization was being used to hasten healing of fractures and burns. We gave it a try.

Under hypnosis, I told Barry the white blood cells were going to invade the area, eating up the bacteria. I told him they were going to break up, releasing enzymes, which would dissolve the dead tissue. I explained that serum would flood the wound, washing out the pus and broken-down tissue. I described how the fibroblasts would multiply, laying down collagen, forming a scar, which would bind the wound edges together.

After I was finished with my description of how to heal an abscess, I brought him out of his trance. He said that of all the crazy things he had done under hypnosis this seemed most strange. It seemed as if his entire being was concentrated on the wound and incision.

By that evening, the wound was no longer swollen, tender, or red! Clear, straw-colored serum was pouring out of the incision. I'm talking about a flood! He had bandages, towels, and the bed soaked. When he stood, a couple of ounces would splash onto the floor, as if poured from a cup. The next day, the serum was still flowing, with no sign of letting up. Barry asked me to hypnotize him and find out what had gone wrong.

So back into trance.

"What's with all the serum?" I asked.

"You told me to,"—and I certainly had. It was like the sorcerer's apprentice, the brooms filling the cistern with water and no command to stop. The serum was washing out the wound, and I had not foreseen the need to tell it when to quit.

"That's true," I replied, "but it has done its job. Now, it needs to stop. Then the wound edges will fall together, the scar will form and heal the incision, and you can go home."

"OK," Barry said in a matter-of-fact voice.

Within twenty minutes, the wound was dry! There was not one drop of serum on the dressing. The following day, the wound edges were firmly sealed, and I discharged him. Twenty-four hours later, he was off on a 100-mile bike trip that he had planned before the surgery. When he returned in a few days, I removed his stitches in the office.

This case demonstrates not only the usefulness of hypnosis as a tool but the power of the mind over the body and its functions. What is hard to comprehend is that this influence of mind over body takes place every day, with everyone. We just don't normally use hypnosis and see the result laid out in the open for our inspection. The cells composing our bodies constantly conform and adjust according to our conscious and subconscious desires and directives. We create our problems in the same way I unwittingly created the flood of serum. We literally get what we ask for.

It follows that we need to become very attentive of our thoughts and ideas. If we become ill, we should carefully examine our core beliefs concerning illness. Many times, we may actually be seeking illness, for one reason or another, and be totally unaware of the directions we have given our bodies. I'm not suggesting, in any fashion, that we should worry about every twinge or feel and poke around for something wrong. That's the worst thing we can do. However, at some point, we need to analyze just what sort of plan we have for our physical being. We need to give our bodies clear, unequivocal directions, outlining the goals we wish to attain.

Not everything I tried with hypnosis worked that well. Barry told me that he had read some articles on obesity that indicated if the person held a mental image of himself as thin he would grow to match the image. I decided to try it. I had a young man in my practice who was very obese. He was also a good hypnotic subject. I suggested he let me hypnotize him and give him a suggestion that he would see himself weighing a normal 180 pounds. He readily agreed. I hypnotized him and suggested that every time he looked into a mirror he would see himself weighing 180. I had him open his eyes and gaze in the mirror while he was hypnotized. He smiled and agreed that he looked great. I suggested that he would eat in such a way that his body would conform to the image in the mirror.

It did not work. He did not lose an ounce. I forgot all about it. Several years later, he asked if I could hypnotize him again. I told him that I would and asked the purpose. He said that when he looked in the mirror he still saw himself as if he weighed 180.

"What's wrong with that?" I asked.

"Well, the only time I could remember weighing 180 was when I was in high school and all I ever wore in high school was a T-shirt and jeans. No matter what I have on, I see myself wearing a T-shirt and jeans, and it's hard to tie my tie when I get dressed to go to work."

The young man had enjoyed his appearance and had held onto his weight and the suggestion in spite of the inconvenience it caused. I hypnotized him and removed the suggestion that he would see himself thin, as he requested. The pity is that if I had known then what I know now, it would have worked. At that time, I had no knowledge of the importance of addressing the bio-consciousness in addition to having the patient "appear" normal in his own eyes. Unless the bio-consciousness is instructed to follow the new suggestions, it will continue in its old pattern.

Years ago, a study was done at Duke University in which researchers interviewed people in the coronary care unit who had sustained heart attacks. In virtually every case, the patient had sought an illness, not necessarily a heart attack in specific, but something. Every patient had some situation from which he wished to escape. Illness was viewed as an acceptable way out—an excuse for a rest, avoiding some project, a respite from a demanding home situation, something. The bio-consciousness had complied with the patient's subconscious wishes.

One hears that people will accept almost any suggestion given to them while they are under hypnosis. For this reason, it is believed the information received is often information implanted by the hypnotist rather than actually coming from the subject. My experience has been the opposite. The hypnotized person does not surrender his or her will, intelligence, integrity, or control simply because of the hypnotic state. Hypnotized individuals are in a state of altered consciousness, not asleep or in limbo. They are aware of their surroundings and in full command. What they do is to accept suggestions made by the hypnotist, providing the suggestions seem appropriate and are to their liking. This, too, is a form of control.

Years ago, I was doing some hypnotherapy with a man who was having a terrible time enjoying any kind of meaningful relationship with his mother. His memories were full of resentment, and he was convinced that his mother had never loved him. I thought that some early recall might give him some new basis for a better relationship. Under hypnosis, I asked him to go back to his birth. I asked him to recall being placed in his mother's arms for the first time.

"My mother doesn't love me," he stated.

"Sure she does," I countered. "Every mother loves her baby."

"I appreciate what you are trying to do, but she doesn't love me. The nurse tried to give me to my mother and she refused to hold me. She told the nurse to 'get the damned kid' out of her sight. She wanted a girl and not a boy."

I tried in vain to convince the man that his mother did not mean what he had heard her say. He was in a deep trance, but he was not buying any suggestion I had to give. He knew better.

During World War II, some psychologist working at an Ivy League university set up an experiment trying to prove a person could be tricked into committing a crime using hypnosis. He selected a Jewish graduate student and hypnotized him. While hypnotized the student was told that Adolf Hitler was asleep in the adjoining room. It was suggested that he would be doing the world a favor by killing Hitler. The subject was then given a loaded pistol and led to the next room where he proceeded to shoot a dummy in the bed full of holes. The conclusion was that anyone could have been in the bed and that the subject could therefore have been duped into murdering someone the hypnotist wished to kill.

Hypnosis

The experiment was full of flaws. First of all, one does not surrender one's brain just because one is hypnotized. Logically, the student knew Hitler was not visiting the United States and certainly would not be sleeping in the psychology laboratory, even if he were. In the second place, it didn't make sense that a boy would be handed a gun to shoot someone in a psych laboratory, not even the head of the department. This was a stage play and nothing more, put on under hypnosis. The student recognized it for what it was and acted out his part in the play.

To further illustrate this point, I was once asked by one of the service clubs in Champaign to speak on hypnosis. In order to discredit those of us who were using hypnosis, a doctor from one of the clinics had been making the rounds, speaking at the various clubs, telling how dangerous hypnosis was. He put out all the usual misinformation doctors use to discreetly disparage one another. I had been invited to give testimony to the opposite side of the question. To make certain I would have someone with whom I could demonstrate hypnosis, I took along a nurse I knew to be an excellent subject.

It was a dinner meeting. They served a very thin, tired slice of roast beef. I turned to the nurse and asked her if she would prefer a T-bone steak. Telling her she was the only one in the room to enjoy a steak, I had her close her eyes. I took about fifteen seconds to hypnotize her and suggested she would be eating a delicious, tender, medium rare T-bone. She opened her eyes and attacked her "steak" sawing off thin slices of beef as if she were cutting into an inch-thick T-bone. She said it was delicious.

When it came time for my speech, I told them what I knew about hypnosis and then placed the nurse into a trance. Among other demonstrations, I stuck 18-gauge needles into her arms and suspended her between two chairs. The audience was impressed. So was I. I had never suspended anyone between a couple of chairs before. Then I asked her if she would like to pretend something. She agreed. She was still hypnotized. I told her I had brought along a trick knife, like ones used in the movies. I explained it would take an expert to tell it was a trick knife, for it looked exactly like a real one. I suggested we put on a little play in which she was to stab me in the chest with the trick knife. Then I produced a hunting knife from my coat. The sucker had an eight-inch blade. Several members of the audience gasped. I handed it to her and at the same time reinforced the suggestion that it was a trick knife and she could not possibly hurt me with it. I told her I would not lie to her and to go on and stab me in the chest. She took the knife and raised it to stab me. She hesitated and I urged her to stab away, telling her it was a fake knife, it only looked and felt real, that I was telling her the truth and I would not be hurt. In a flash, she came out of her trance proclaiming it was real, not a fake, and demanded to know why I was lying to her. I rest my case.

Hypnosis is a valid, useful tool, which can be used widely in all areas of medicine. During deep trance states the subconscious mind is able to tap into the spiritual memory that transcends physical existence. As with any method that might be used to dredge up old, forgotten memories, one needs to use prudence and judgment. Defenses cannot be stripped away from painful events. The patient must be respected and handled with skill.

Of course, hypnosis can be used by unscrupulous and misguided therapists to implant false concepts in the minds of their patients. The same thing can be accomplished with any form of counseling or therapy. If a therapist is working with a mixed up, spiritually disturbed patient and keeps insisting that certain things are so, the patient can be brainwashed into accepting almost anything as true. There is a tendency to blame the use of hypnosis for these unfortunate results rather than the therapist. Such condemnation by association is never warranted.

Some of the case histories I have related were a bit more involved than they appear here. I simplified the stories, making them less cluttered so the relevant points would be more easily appreciated.

In spite of the need for some talent and skill in counseling and dealing with emotional problems, hypnosis should be high on the list of useful investigational and therapeutic methods. In my opinion every physician should be as skilled in the use of hypnosis as he is with his stethoscope.

SUGGESTIONS
AND SURGERY

URING MY INTERNSHIP and, later, during my surgical residency, I was under the training of two of Chicago's best surgeons. I would do the history and physical on each surgical patient on admission, assist in surgery as the first or second assistant, and monitor postoperative care while the patients remained in the hospital. When each patient was discharged, I would stand about while the surgeon gave him or her instructions concerning postoperative care and activity. Usually this consisted of a long list of things not to do. The patient was not to lift, climb stairs, drive an automobile, bathe, eat certain things, and, definitely, not return to work for a period of time. After an intra-abdominal operation or a hernia repair, this time of imposed inactivity usually ranged from four to six weeks. It was all very standard and very accepted. Every surgeon gave patients essentially the same instructions.

I was always intrigued by the patients who refused to obey the doctor and did what they pleased. I used to hope secretly that something would go wrong, just to prove to the patient that the surgeon knew best—but nothing *ever* went wrong. About the time I started practice, I read a couple of articles in which surgeons were advocating immediate ambulation and a return to normal activities. It occurred to me that those patients who flagrantly disregarded the commands to do nothing and avoid activity were probably instinctively doing the right thing. I concluded that was why they never got into trouble.

In the preceding chapter, I told how I learned that people could hear even though they were asleep with a general anesthetic. In fact, people do not lose their hearing even when unconscious with a head injury or in a coma from an illness. One man was brought to the hospital during my internship with a severe head injury. He lay unconscious in a two-bed ward for about three weeks. One day after he had regained consciousness and was able to speak, he said something about being in the hospital a long time. Trying to ease the truth, I remarked it wasn't all that long. He countered by saying there had been five patients in the other bed since he arrived. He even remembered their names and what had been wrong with each of them. The nurse and I didn't believe him, so we checked the patient logbook. Sure enough, he was absolutely right on every count. Most people cannot consciously remember what took place when they were in a coma or under a general anesthetic. However, under hypnosis, people can recount vividly events occurring in their rooms while they were supposedly unconscious.

An orthopedic surgeon referred a patient who had a back problem. She had been operated on by another surgeon and, although he had gotten the operative report, it was unclear just what had been found. He thought that, under hypnosis, the patient might be able to shed some light on the matter, providing she could recall what was said during the operation. My friend was a good, honest surgeon and was also troubled by the patient's apparent unwillingness to trust him fully. Actually, she was almost hostile toward him, and he had done nothing to her.

Under hypnosis, the patient vividly recalled what she had heard. During the operation, the surgeon did not find a ruptured disc. She heard her family doctor, who was assisting in the surgery, arguing with the orthopedic surgeon as to whether they had even operated on the correct disc. The surgeon confessed he didn't think she even had a ruptured disc. Furthermore, he said some surgeon would eventually operate on her so he might as well get the money as the next guy. Then the two got together, cooking up a story to tell, so they would not cross each other up. By the time the lady related this, she was swearing and so angry that she could hardly talk. Little wonder the woman was having a hard time trusting doctors.

All sorts of frightening and terrible things are said in the operating room when a patient is anesthetized. The remarks are particularly frightening when heard by a patient who is not used to normal medical jargon or familiar with how doctors speak to one another. Perfectly innocent statements are frequently interpreted as ominous and accepted by the subconscious mind as a core belief to be passed on to the cells.

Then statements are made that are not so benign, such as the case of the lady we just mentioned. It is not unusual for the surgeon to inquire of the anesthetist if the patient is asleep and then make all sorts of nasty, personal comments about the patient. I heard one doctor refer to his patient as a "God damned fat bitch." He had no idea the patient was hearing every insulting word.

Anesthesia ordinarily produces amnesia so that, upon awakening, the patient cannot consciously recall what he or she has heard. But it's all there, stored in the subconscious. After surgery, the doctor may wonder why the patient no longer seems so friendly. One cannot help wondering how many malpractice suits are fostered by a patient's subconscious desire to get even with the surgeon who insulted him.

An incident occurred to me when I was fourteen. My family and I were on vacation and had stopped to see my uncle, the doctor in Kansas, when I developed acute appendicitis. I was put to sleep with ether. As I was being anesthetized, I could hear the clatter of instruments, and suddenly I was aware of my uncle's voice saying

"Scalpel—clamp—sponge—." I realized that they were operating on me! Then, I lost consciousness. Later, I told my uncle about it, and he said that I had imagined it all.

After reading articles that patients under anesthesia respond to suggestions as if they were hypnotized, and based upon my own experiences that early activity is helpful in stimulating wound healing and preventing complications, I launched into a program to determine whether I could alter postoperative recovery by giving suggestions during surgery, while the patient was asleep. Before starting this program, I had made it a practice to play music to my patients through headphones. The purpose was to keep them from hearing inadvertent remarks, which might be frightening or misunderstood. Then, I realized that I was missing the whole point. Rather than masking their hearing, I should use it.

I knew that, for this to be effective, there had to be a three-pronged approach involving the preoperative, operative, and postoperative periods. Suggestions begin in the office, when the possibility of surgery is being discussed, as well as in the hospital. All patients contemplating surgery inquire about three things: Will they be all right? Will they suffer? How soon will they be back to normal? To these questions, I told my patients to expect a short, pleasant hospitalization. I impressed upon them that how much discomfort they would have was totally up to them. What is more, I explained the process of wound healing, telling them that the more they moved about, the more quickly the scar would form and the stronger it would be. To the question of when they would be all right again, they were told they could leave the hospital in a day or two and return to work immediately, if they so wished. Sometimes, a patient would tell me about his Aunt Tillie who had a terrible time with her gallbladder surgery. My reply was that I had not been her doctor and these things I was telling them were true because I would use magic to heal them. With this approach, my patients entered the hospital with the idea that theirs was to be a unique and pleasant experience.

The next arena was the operating room itself. Everyone was instructed that the patient could hear everything taking place and being said. Therefore, they were to say nothing they would not say if the patient were awake. I even posted signs on the door instructing the nurses and doctors to watch their language. But I could never break the pathologist from making stupid remarks. For that reason, my experimental group of cases did not include breast surgery for cancer. The pathologist would come to the operating room after examining the biopsy and make statements such as, "Well, she's had it. The lymph nodes are involved. She'll be dead inside a year." My breast cases were all depressed after surgery.

Once the OR was "cleaned" of inappropriate remarks, I talked to the patients as surgery was being performed, telling them things were going fine, that there was nothing we did not expect. I'd tell them how much better they were going to feel. If some remark was made that might be misunderstood, I'd explain in lay terms what had been said. If an instrument was dropped and someone said "oops," I would tell the patients what had occurred. As the operations neared completion I would explain exactly what had been done and give the patients a list of instructions for their bodies. I would tell them how much better they were going to feel now that their diseased organs had been removed, or whatever was appropriate to the surgery performed. They were told that they would be hungry and have their normal appetites—moreover, that we had done nothing to interfere with the normal workings of their intestines or urinary bladders. They were instructed to move about freely, thereby stimulating wound healing and preventing the incisions from feeling sore and stiff. They were told the incisions would heal quickly, without swelling, infection, or tenderness. They were to sleep soundly in their normal natural positions. They were also told they could go home the next day if they desired and return to work immediately. I gave every suggestion I could think of that would help the postoperative course. (And, no, I never had the nerve to suggest they pay their bill promptly.)

My anesthetist cooperated fully. She would have the patients awake and talking to us as they were wheeled to the recovery room. We gave no preoperative sedatives, so, once the anesthetic was out of the system, the patients were fully alert.

After the patients returned to their rooms, the same positive attitude was carried forth by the nurses on the floor. They were to refrain from asking the patients if they wanted anything for pain. Instead, they were to ask only if there was anything they could do for them. They were not to decide whether the patients needed a bedpan. They were to wait until the patients said they needed to urinate, and then take them to the bathroom.

The results were outstanding. If I had done an eight o'clock gallbladder, it was the usual thing for the patient to be eating a regular diet at noon. I never had a single patient with postoperative nausea or a distended abdomen from intestinal ileus. The patients urinated without being catheterized, and this included hysterectomies. These were not minor cases. They included gastric resections, bowel and colon surgery, cholecystectomies, with or without common duct explorations, total abdominal hysterectomies, appendectomies, and hernia repairs. Naturally, I did not have a gastric resection eating dinner the day of surgery. There were some variations, depending upon the surgery performed.

I published a paper on the positive effect of suggestion on the postoperative recovery of surgical patients.

Ruth was a typical case. She had large, double-inguinal hernias and needed a hysterectomy because of bleeding fibroid tumors. I operated on her, doing a total hysterectomy, including both tubes and ovaries. Then, through two more incisions, I repaired the hernias. She had three incisions. She ate a full meal at noon, and when I made rounds late that evening, I found her curled up, lying on her stomach, sound asleep, in her "normal natural position."

The next morning when I made rounds she was not in her room. She was up walking around the hospital, visiting with friends, and other patients with whom she was acquainted. On the second day, she asked to go home, saying it was a shame to take up bed space when she didn't need it. I discharged her, told her to do what she felt like, and gave her an appointment to come to the office to remove her stitches.

Ruth's husband was at work. Since she had driven herself to the hospital, she drove home. Upon arriving home, she found she needed some groceries, so she drove to the store to do her weekly shopping. Coming out of the store with a bag of groceries in each arm, she met a friend. The friend wanted to know why her surgery had been canceled. Ruth assured her it had not and, as proof, pulled down the top of her skirt to expose the incision. Her friend fainted dead away.

Ruth was laughing as she related the story to me when I was removing her skin stitches. She said she hadn't figured on having to lift her friend off the sidewalk and help her into her car. Ruth was fine and her incisions were solidly healed.

These things were not accomplished without some difficulty and interference by my colleagues. One of my patients was in a four-bed ward. It was her first day following surgery, and she was doing very well, eating a general diet and walking about all over the hospital. Another doctor, a board-certified surgeon, had a patient on whom he had performed an identical operation several days before. His patient had not been allowed to eat a full diet and was not yet walking. She must have asked him why she could not be doing what my patient was doing. Suddenly, I heard him saying loudly, for everyone in the entire ward to hear, that she was not to listen to what I told my patient, for I was foolhardy and dangerous. He predicted I would get into trouble some day with my outlandish practices, and he was personally going to enjoy helping put me in my place. My patient, a long-time acquaintance, winked at me. I returned the wink and we enjoyed the joke. Later, she asked if what the doctor had done was not unethical. I told her it was but that we nonconformists are fair game for anyone who comes along wanting to take potshots at us.

I took one man's gallbladder out and sent him home on the second day after surgery. On the seventh day, he came to the office to have his stitches removed. He had been washing windows and putting up storm windows for the preceding two days and wanted to know if he could return to work. He said he had been more active than if he had been on the job.

The power of the mind is almost beyond imagination. We simply have to make certain it is directed toward health and not disease. The mind can be used to facilitate healing in other settings besides surgery through the process of talking to the cells and giving specific directions. Fractures heal more promptly if the patient spends fifteen minutes or so every day visualizing the healing process. It is not important to understand how bones heal. If he so desires, the patient can imagine little elves laying down bricks of bone to bridge the injury. The important thing is the atmosphere of positive intent produced by the process. In contrast, the person who stares at his broken leg—hating his predicament, imagining his terrible luck and all manner of bad things happening to him—may well delay the healing or even cause the fracture *not* to heal. In these cases, the attitude and thoughts concerning failure and bad luck become instructions to the cells not to heal.

There are a number of things any patient can do to facilitate her recovery from surgery, even if the doctor does not give positive suggestions as I did. Understand that your subconscious mind will not let you hurt yourself if you use a bit of common sense. It is a proven fact that wounds heal faster and stronger if the patient is active, so return to normal activity as soon as possible. If your nutrition is poor, wound healing may be delayed, so take your vitamin-mineral supplement. Last, and possibly most important, talk to your body. Tell it to do what it needs to accomplish rapid healing and recovery. The cells know how to heal themselves if we leave them alone and do not confuse the issue with contradictory instructions in the form of fears and other destructive thoughts. Keep a positive attitude. Your body knows how to heal itself. It does not need instruction from the doctor. Get in a quiet place and picture your body taking command. Imagine all the forces of healing joining together and returning everything to normal. After babies and dogs are operated upon, it is impossible for anyone to keep them quiet. They are moving and jumping about all over the place. Their wounds do not fall apart.

It is not uncommon for the doctor to aid the destructive forces preventing recovery. This is purely unintentional, for no doctor wants this to happen. What has developed over the years is a whole change in attitude of both the patients and the doctors through a number of changes taking place in society. One huge area of change is the increase in malpractice suits.

I know one surgeon who takes great pains to tell his patients it may be weeks before they recover and regain their strength. He tells them they will have pain, gas, and all manner of unpleasant things. He paints a very bleak picture of the postoperative course. This man is a good surgeon as far as the surgical technique goes, but you know what? His patients take weeks to recover and usually experience all the things he suggests to them. My guess is he figures that if the patient has a rough time postoperatively then the patient can't say he wasn't warned; if not, then the doctor was marvelous and the patient is happy. Unfortunately, most patients hear remarks of this kind as commands. The surgeon is a powerful person, so the patient feels obliged to comply. It reminds me of the joke that is actually so true it is frightening: "He's a good doctor. What he says you got, that's what you die of."

An obstetrician I knew had a very high C-section rate. Patient after patient would start into labor and, after a few hours, the contractions would lose their strength and labor would come to a slow halt. Medicine to stimulate the labor contractions often failed. After a while, depending on whether the membranes had ruptured or how dilated the cervix was, there was no recourse but to do a section.

It is a physiological fact that anxiety tends to produce hormones within the body that stop or delay labor. In some animal species, the female can delay labor for hours or days if the environment in which to deliver the young safely is not present. The same hormones are present in people.

It was amazing to watch and listen to this particular doctor in the presence of his patients in labor. He obviously had very little confidence in his ability and was scared to death that something might happen for which he would be blamed. He hovered over his patients from the moment they entered the hospital. He was visibly worried to the point of appearing frantic. He fussed over every contraction, asking the nurse if she thought labor was stopping. He checked the fetal monitor, questioning aloud whether it was working properly. He constantly talked about the possible need to do a section. All this took place in the birthing room, creating an atmosphere of fear and anxiety. No wonder labor stopped!

A huge problem, not unrelated to the subject of suggestion, is that we have become the most litigious society in history. We can't walk down the street and stub a toe without looking about for someone to blame and sue. No one seems willing to assume responsibility for his or her own actions or destiny. The legal profession, which may be the only profession as greedy as the medical profession, has encouraged this mad rush to court. Its members have silently inserted themselves between every doctor and every patient in every situation. There is not a single physician who does not fear a frivolous suit. And there no longer need be any real grounds for a claim. Anything short of a perfect result will more than likely lead to a malpractice suit, whether the doctor had anything to do with the result or not. There is always an unscrupulous attorney ready to file a suit, knowing the insurance company will settle for a few thousand dollars simply to get the case settled. Naturally, the attorney pockets at least half of the settlement just for writing a few letters.

With this change of climate, doctors have become fearful of reassuring the patient. Suits have actually been filed and won when a doctor, in an effort to comfort the patient, has told him or her not to worry, that things would be all right. Such statements have been taken by the courts as a contract to cure. When the patient did not recover according to his or her expectations, the doctor was sued for breach of contract. Whether these cases are rare or commonplace is irrelevant. Physicians hear about them, and malpractice is constantly in their thoughts, causing most to run tests endlessly in an attempt to protect themselves. Of course, some doctors frighten more easily than others, but the facts are that the vast majority have been sued and all too many of those cases have been unfounded. They may involve a poor result, but the poor result is often the fault of no one—or even the fault of the patient. Noncompliance on the part of the patient is extremely common: not taking medicine, not following instructions. Often, the emotional attitude of the patient affects the outcome of the healing process. The legal system has bought the concept that getting well is entirely under the control of the doctor. If a patient does not return to exactly the way she was prior to an injury or illness, does it truly follow that it must be the fault of the doctor?

As a consequence, doctors are less and less apt to comfort, reassure or even talk to their patients. It's hard to twist the doctor's meaning if the doctor says nothing. People tend to hear what they want to hear. When the doctor remarks she will treat a patient or see what can be done, the patient often "hears" that he will be cured or taken care of. The consequences of these meanings are vastly different.

It would be to everyone's best interest to avoid reading into statements a meaning not there. One good way to avoid this is to repeat back to the doctor what you believe she said. I'm sure more conversation would follow and better communication would result. I've had patients insist I told them things so bizarre that I could not imagine what I might have said that could have been so twisted around.

My first encounter with this phenomenon occurred during my internship. A lady was admitted to the hospital for thyroid surgery the following day. It was my job to do a complete history and physical exam the evening of admission. Part of the exam was to do a pelvic examination. Other than her thyroid, the physical exam was normal, except for a small cervical erosion. Now, cervical "erosion" is a poor term. It only has the appearance of being eroded and is an extremely common finding of no importance. She asked if everything was normal and I assured her it was. Then I added she had a small cervical erosion of no consequence and nothing to worry about.

Then she wanted to know if the surgeon would attend to it at the same time he did her thyroid surgery? I told her I doubted it, but she should discuss it with him. She asked if he did not attend to it, who would? I answered it did not really need to be attended to by anyone, but if he thought it did he would probably do it at another time or refer her to another doctor. Again, I suggested she take it up with the surgeon. That was the end of the conversation.

Some weeks later, the surgeon came to me, mad as a hornet. He demanded to know why I would say such a thing to the patient. She claimed I had told her she had a far advanced cancer of the cervix, and that he was going to refer her to Dr. _____ , who was a gynecologist. He was supposed to have done this while she was in the hospital. She was angry for his having ignored her cancer all those weeks. I did my best to defend myself, but I doubt the surgeon ever believed me.

Patients often claim that surgeons do not explain things or tell them about complications or even what was done. Several years ago, a cardiovascular surgeon published an article on this very subject. He secretly tape recorded his preoperative conversation with each patient the evening before surgery. He would identify himself by name, as well as have the patient state his or her name. Then, he would carefully explain what was to be done, the possible complications, the risks, the whole works. He did this with a large number of patients.

A year later, he mailed each of them a questionnaire. Did the surgeon see you before surgery? Did he talk with you? Did he tell you what he was to do? Did he explain the risks and possible complications? One third of the patients recalled the visit and conversation with fair detail. One third remembered his visit but recalled very little of what had been said. The final third stated flatly that the surgeon had not seen them prior to surgery nor had he told them anything at all concerning the operation, possible complications, or anything whatsoever. When the tape recordings were played back to them, they denied the voices being theirs, even when they heard themselves stating their own names.

This is not surprising. Often, after spending twenty or thirty minutes with a patient, explaining things and answering questions, he or she would call back, complaining to my nurse that I had explained nothing and spent no time talking. This is more apt to happen with mothers and kids. Lots of pediatricians give printed instructions because it is common for parents to hear nothing of what is said in the office.

Explanations are often taken as suggestions. It is through communication that surgeons, like medical doctors, exert much of their most potent and lasting effects. As I have said, thoughts are things as real as rocks. Suggestions accepted by the patient, whether they come from the surgeon, arise within the patient, or are implanted by relatives or friends, are frequently incorporated into the patient's belief system. And, thus, they affect the outcome of every illness, treatment, and surgical procedure.

THE PROBLEMS
WITH PATIENTS

THROUGHOUT THIS BOOK, I have been very critical of physicians. My observations concerning their attitudes and shortcomings are valid, but the patients are active partners in everything the physician does. There is an East Indian saying that when the hands are clapped, both hands take part in the clapping. In the case of healing, there may be more than one set of hands. In our rush to place blame on the medical profession for all that goes wrong, we must not forget that each patient comes to the doctor with a complaint. The doctor did not go out into the street and drag in a healthy, happy person and start running tests and prescribing treatments. *The doctor is never responsible for the patient's original problem.* On occasion, the physician may contribute to the problem but he or she is never responsible for the original complaint of the patient.

An old Navy Commander taught me this lesson when I was stationed at the US Navy Hospital at Camp LeJeune, North Carolina. He was the Chief of Surgery, and I was a ward surgeon under his command. A Chief Petty Officer was admitted to have a tendon repair done on his ring finger. He had cut the flexor tendon while making toys in the hobby shop for his kids for Christmas and had been treated in sick bay for almost two weeks before being referred to the hospital. The battalion surgeon, a dermatologist who knew nothing about hand injuries and just didn't know any better, had procrastinated sending him to the hospital. By the time I saw the Chief, his finger was stiff as a post and there was a large, infected hole over the place where the tendon had been cut. To make a long story short, after two months in the hospital and three different operations he still did not have a serviceable finger. To be honest, every attempt to heal the infection and graft a new tendon had failed. I felt badly and somewhat responsible for the situation. The Chief was also depressed and obviously unhappy.

One morning, the Commander made rounds with me, and afterward we sat and talked. One of the points of discussion was the miserable results I had had with the Chief. All my other hand cases and tendon grafts were getting along beautifully. One thing that made it so hard for me to accept was that I was sincerely fond of the Chief.

The Commander looked at me and said, "You feel pretty badly about the results on the Chief's finger, don't you, Bonnett? You sort of feel responsible for it all."

"Well, yes, I do. Everything I have tried has failed. This last time I lost the pedicle graft because of a reaction to the Furacin ointment dressings."

"You blame yourself for it all happening, do you?"

"Well, I guess I do," I admitted.

"From the way the Chief was acting, it is clear that he blames you, too." The Commander's eyes were boring into mine.

"I can hardly blame him," I replied.

"Tell me, did you shove the Chief's hand into that saw and cut his finger?"

"Of course not."

"I think the Chief has forgotten that and you have, too. Now, tomorrow, when you make rounds, you can be as nice and sympathetic as you want, just like you have been all along. But before you leave his bedside, I want you to say to him, 'It sure is a shame you had to cut your finger in that saw.'"

"That's silly."

"No, that's a command from me to you."

The next morning, I did as he commanded. The Chief's mouth dropped open, and he just stared at me. Later in the day, the Chief came into my office. He thanked me for my efforts in trying to save the use of his finger. Then he said, "Look, Doc, you've done your best. Why don't you cut the damn thing off in the morning so I can get back to duty?"

And that is what I did. For years, I got a Christmas card from him thanking me for my efforts and for taking care of him. I had forgotten that I had not been responsible for the predicament. I hadn't cut his finger. The Chief had done it all by himself. I have always been thankful to Dr. Lawler for the valuable lesson he taught me that day, over a cup of coffee in my office.

This anecdote brings us to the general subject of patient responsibility. Whether you choose to call it health care or the treatment of illness, it is a cooperative adventure between the physician, the patient, his relatives, the hospital personnel, the legal profession, government agencies, and society in general. The public has allowed, and in some instances invited, all these various individuals and agents to come between the patient and his doctor. If this is what the patient wants, so be it, but then she cannot expect to have the close personal relationship with her doctor that used to occur in her grandparents' day. Arguments could be made that many medical changes over the past two generations have been for the good. On the other hand, healing is a very personal event, and if the doctor is to be a healer and not just a skilled technician, anything that intrudes between him and the patient necessarily lessens the effectiveness of both their efforts.

One of the attitudes of patients that is central to the problem is that of unreasonable expectation. I have had patients express shock when I mentioned where the scar was going to be after their surgery. They stated they did not know they were going to have a scar. It was not as though they had never seen an operative scar on someone. How can the surgeon cut into the body, sew it up, and the body heal without the formation of a scar? Such an attitude is complete denial of reality and in opposition to common sense. No reasonable person can expect to break arms and legs, be torn up in accidents of various types, survive illnesses and diseases that would have been fatal twenty years ago, and expect, every time, to be exactly the same as before the event. Usually, things turn out pretty well, but when they do not, it is not automatically the fault of the doctor.

One of my orthopedic friends attended a man who had been in a motorcycle accident. One could argue that the patient was totally responsible, for he entered the emergency room roaring drunk with a blood alcohol level of 2.4. He had sustained multiple fractures of his leg. The injury was so severe that there were nineteen separate bone fragments in his lower leg. Two of the fracture lines extended into the knee joint. In addition to the fractures, there was a massive injury to the soft tissues, the muscles, and skin. He was lucky to save the man's leg at all. For his efforts, he was sued because the man's knee was stiff, he did not have a full range of motion, and he walked with a limp. Members of the jury said later that they awarded the man a half-million dollars not because they believed the doctor had mishandled the case but because they felt sorry for the patient.

Many patients expect immediate results from the medicine they take. When treating an infection, a strep throat for example, the antibiotic will kill the majority of the disease bacteria in the first few hours. But before the patient will experience any relief of symptoms, the body has to do a number of things. The toxins produced by the germs have to be removed from the throat tissues and neutralized by the body. Dead and dying cells have to be cleared from the area. Swelling must go down, and many other things must occur before the temperature returns to normal and the pain in the throat muscles subsides. I made it a practice of telling my patients that it would be at least forty-eight hours before they would feel any better. In spite of my statement, it was common for the patient, or a parent, to call my home that evening angrily complaining that there had been no improvement. These patients had taken, at the most, two or three doses of the antibiotic, and no more than five or six hours had passed. One woman called after giving her child one spoonful of antibiotic, claiming that the medicine was not working. Time is required for the body to heal itself. Medicines do not heal. No medicine has ever healed anything. People heal.

Often, the patient is responsible for an unwanted result simply for failing to follow advice. Many times, patients fail to return for much needed visits that would allow the doctor an opportunity to monitor the course of the treatment. An orthopedic surgeon under whom I trained treated a man with a broken leg. After applying the cast, he instructed the patient to use crutches and to return in a week. That was the last time he saw the fellow until a year later when he was in court being sued by the patient. The man had suffered a horrible result and, as evidence of his bad care, his lawyers displayed an ill-fitting cast. On the witness stand, the doctor said, "That is not the cast I applied. The patient did not return to me for follow-up visits, and I am not responsible for the result. The doctor who applied that particular cast is responsible." The lawyer insisted it *was* the cast the doctor had applied and that there had been no other doctor. To this, my friend countered that there was no cartoon of Mickey Mouse on the cast. He explained that he always drew a Mickey Mouse on every cast he applied, and, since this one did not have the cartoon, it was not his. The lawsuit was dismissed. If it had not been for a missing Mickey Mouse, the lies of the patient might have held up.

As I said earlier, patients frequently fail to listen to the doctor. I have had patients claim I did not ask them to return, even when they had made a return appointment before leaving the office.

In an earlier chapter, I told about a study revealing that patients often fail to recall that the doctor talked with them before their surgery. I gave another example with the woman who claimed I had told her she had a cancer of the cervix, when I had said no such thing. In that instance, she was projecting her own fears onto my words. It probably would not have mattered what I had said to her; she was expecting to hear that she had a cancer.

Rarely do patients take the medicine that is prescribed in the full amounts or at the proper times. One bizarre case I had involved a new patient who came to see me complaining of some abdominal discomfort. I examined him and told the man that I felt he had a spastic colon. I gave him a prescription and asked him to return in one week. The day before his return appointment, I happened to be in one of the drugstores visiting with the pharmacist. On a shelf were four or five dozen bottles of medicine that had not been picked up. There in front of me on one of the bottles, I noticed my name and the medicine I had prescribed for the man with the spastic colon. He had given the prescription to the pharmacist but had not returned to get it. The pharmacist said that was a common occurrence.

I certainly did not expect the man to return, but the next day he showed up for his appointment.

"How are you feeling today?" I asked.

"I'm not a bit better. The God-damned medicine wasn't any good."

"It can't help if you don't take it," I countered.

"What do you mean?"

"You never picked the medicine up. It's still in Skelton's drugstore. I can understand why you might have decided not to take the medicine, but I can't reason why you would come back to me to complain about medicine you didn't take. If you did not have any confidence in me or the diagnosis, that's one thing, but why did you bother to return?"

"The stuff wouldn't have helped anyway!" he responded angrily.

"I don't have time to waste on people like you," I growled. "Get the hell out of my office, and find someone else to play your games with." Needless to say, he left.

This brings up another subject. Patients commonly do not tell the doctor the truth, or at least not all of it. A classic example was demonstrated by Kit when I inquired as to whether Carl was creeping, walking, and talking (*see* page 83). She was worried, and it was easier to lie to me than face her fear at that moment. It was only when threatened by the diagnoses of the other doctors that she realized she had to admit the problem.

When asked if they are taking medicine from the drugstore or from another doctor, often patients will deny it. Sometimes, patients are seeing two different physicians and taking medicine from both. If they happen to take the prescriptions to the same drugstore, the computer will identify this information and the pharmacist will inform the doctors. If the patient goes to different pharmacies, there is little chance that the duplication of medicines will be discovered, unless the patient has some bad effect from taking conflicting medicines or taking double doses. I had one patient admitted to the hospital with a severe heart block. Laboratory tests revealed he was nearly dead from a massive overdose of digitoxin. The patient managed to survive more by luck than through my skill. Afterward, he admitted that he was going to two other doctors besides me and that we all had prescribed the same medicine. He said his reason was that he believed one single little pill was not enough to do any good and that he needed more medicine than I had given him. He figured out a way to increase his medicine by getting a prescription from us all.

Refusal to believe the doctor knows what he or she is talking about is a problem with occasional patients. One individual I knew was a very stubborn man. His small child had congenital dislocated hips, so he took her to the local children's clinic. There, the surgeon placed the child in a Denny-Brown splint. On her return the next month, the doctor found the child's feet strapped securely in the splint but turned the opposite direction from which he had placed them. The doctor readjusted the splint and told the father not to change the splint in any way. The man took the child home and immediately loosened the splint and reversed the direction. This went on for about six months. At every visit, the doctor showed the father X-rays and articles in an attempt to convince the man that he knew what he was talking about and that the father should leave the splint alone. But the man always stubbornly changed the splints, for he was convinced that he was right and the doctor wrong. Eventually, the doctor removed the splint and instructed the father not to return with the child unless he agreed to cooperate. The end result was that the child remained a cripple. The father enjoyed telling everyone that she was handicapped because the doctor did not know what he was doing.

Families often interfere with a patient's receiving proper care. The case I just related is obvious, but there are times when families, in their concern, start dictating what should and should not be done in a certain situation. More times than not, this is destructive. It usually happens when an out-of-town relative who is never around and has never taken any interest in the welfare of Aunt Tillie comes rushing to the hospital and starts making demands and threats. Any psychologist will tell you that this sort of behavior is an attempt to cover a sense of guilt for neglecting the old lady all those years. The relatives who have been taking care of Aunt Tillie are usually afraid to create a scene, and so they allow the outsider to run amok. The doctor is caught in the middle between his patient, who needs his full attention, and the problems of fending off hostile relatives. In situations where the patient is critically ill and the relatives are giving the physician a hard time, they are sometimes successful in preventing the patient from recovering, or at the least they prolong the recovery time. Trying to treat a person properly when she or he is seriously ill is very difficult in the midst of a family fight. It is the most stressful situation a doctor can be in.

In my practice, I had a lovely old lady who was 89 years old. She was in excellent health for her age and, except for high blood pressure, which was completely controlled with medicine, there was really nothing much wrong with her. In retrospect, she probably had some inkling of what might happen, for she often talked about how she wanted to be treated should she develop a fatal illness. I had recorded her wishes in her office chart. Essentially, she did not wish to be placed on a ventilator or be kept "alive" by means of tubes, machines, and technology. The day came when she had a massive heart attack. She made a remarkable recovery from this event. Still, the relatives were angry, stating that she had not had any heart trouble before and that they could not understand how she could possibly have had a coronary. My explanations were rejected, totally. They appeared to believe nothing I had to say.

On about the sixth day of her recovery, she sustained a stroke. It was a massive, dense stroke that rendered her totally paralyzed on the right side and speechless. At this point, the relatives informed me that if she died they would sue me. Every time I made a hospital visit, one of them was there in the room glaring at me. I would speak pleasantly to them and be met with hostile silence. The old lady refused to eat or drink. She wanted to die. The relatives insisted I place a stomach tube in her so that she could be fed. I explained that this was not her wish. I told them that we had talked about this eventuality and she wanted to be allowed to die rather than be kept alive in that manner. (This was years before living wills and enduring powers of attorney.) Again, I was told that I would be sued if I did not comply with the family's wishes.

So I inserted a feeding tube with the old lady looking daggers at me. I told her that I wanted to respect her wishes but that I had little choice, for her relatives had threatened to sue me if I did not insert the tube. She rolled her eyes, gave a big smile, and quit struggling. A few days later, I transferred her to a nursing home. Three weeks later she sustained another stroke, this time on the left side. She died before she could be transferred back to the hospital.

Patients often do not realize that they may be bringing more than one problem to the doctor when they seek help. In addition to the one they present, there are often other conditions that play a great role in the outcome of the case. One gentleman of my acquaintance went to a surgeon with a problem of circulation in his legs. Those were the days when removing the lumbar sympathetic chain of nerves in the lower abdomen was used to help dilate the blood vessels and improve circulation. The surgeon operated on the man and removed the nerve ganglia. Six days later, the patient's incision fell apart and his bowels protruded to the outside. The difficulty was that the patient had brought a whole list of troubles to the doctor besides his poor circulation. First of all, his nutrition was terrible and he had borderline scurvy. He was also a heavy smoker and had a bad cough. He was an alcoholic, too. The constant coughing, coupled with the malnutrition and alcoholism, had resulted in extremely poor tissue integrity, which cause the man literally to cough his wound apart. When the surgeon operated the second time to sew up his belly, the stitches were intact, but the abdominal wall had split apart, because of the unhealthy tissue. The patient believed that the surgeon had not done a proper job.

Frequently, a patient places constraints on the physician and prevents her from obtaining the tests needed to make an accurate diagnosis and a proper evaluation of the situation. This next case illustrates, in a roundabout fashion, the frustration of the family physician and the problems that result when the patient will not agree to needed tests. The mother of a physician friend, a lady in her late 80s, had a mini-stroke. These are called TIAs, or transient ischemic attacks. Her family doctor examined her and recommended she do nothing other than pay better attention to her mild hypertension and take her medicine more faithfully. Since she had a slight murmur in her neck over the carotid artery, he suggested a number of tests and X-rays, but she declined to have them performed. Her husband insisted she see a local neurosurgeon, for he had read about carotid artery surgery and wanted his wife to have her arteries cleaned out. The local neurosurgeon suggested immediate surgery without benefit of any tests to support his opinion, although I'm sure he would have done a carotid arteriogram before actually attempting the surgery. My friend, though he was a physician, was not in a position to argue with the neurosurgeon. For this reason, he suggested she go to a prestigious clinic in the Midwest to see a famous neurosurgeon there. Her family doctor readily agreed, for he did not think she was a good candidate for the carotid surgery. My friend chartered a plane and took his mother to the "Mecca."

She was examined by a battery of students, interns, and Fellows for several days. Then she was subjected to a barrage of tests and X-rays of all kinds. During all this time she saw neither hide nor hair of the surgeon she had gone to see. Finally, on the day before she was discharged, the famous neurosurgeon came into her room. He said he had gone over her hospital chart and felt that surgery constituted more of a risk than it could possibly do good. He advised her to be more consistent in taking her blood pressure medicine. That was it. No examination; just an opinion based upon the results of the tests and the examination and physical findings of the interns and Fellows—and a bill for some $25,000. Her doctor son reminded his parents that this was the same advice their family doctor had given them. Their response was that the famous clinic had run all those tests and therefore they were more satisfied and glad to have come. They refused to discuss the fact that they had denied their family doctor the privilege of running the same tests that the clinic had run.

My friend remarked to me, "Boy, couldn't we be great doctors if the patients would extend to us the same advantages they extend to the big clinics?" It is true. Often, when tests are suggested, the patient refuses, objecting on the basis of cost or complaining that the testing is inconvenient, or offering one of many other illogical reasons. This does not happen when a patient goes to a university setting. There, it seems, the patient's attitude is, "Here is my body. Do with it what you wish."

For many reasons, some valid and some not, our society has taken the position that we can trust no one—which could be the subject of a book in itself. For whatever the reasons, people do not trust themselves, either. They are afraid to think for themselves, do for themselves, or look out for themselves. We hear it said all the time that a person cannot love others unless he is able to love himself. It is the same for trust. Lack of trust is probably the greatest single factor in people not getting the good medical care they need. They frequently look at the doctor as if he were the enemy. Certainly, there are horror stories about terrible things happening when doctors are inept or unscrupulous. But, dramatic as they may be, they are not the usual cases. These stories have been played up in television programs and news articles because they are sensational. I am aware that I have related a few horror stories of my own, but in most instances, the message was to take charge of your own life, to advise that you not let others lead you blindly about.

In my experience, it was not uncommon for a patient, upon receiving a prescription, to say, "This isn't going to hurt me, is it?" Some even threw the prescriptions back on my desk and left when I would not guarantee that they would suffer no side effects. On occasion, I wanted to snap back, "That's the whole idea. The first pill you swallow is designed to kill you. I kill all my patients by giving them medicine."

Side effects in themselves are an interesting subject. Some years ago the *New England Journal of Medicine* published a paper on "non-drug reactions." Some doctors had interviewed 300 or 400 hospital employees who said they had not been ill during the preceding three days and had not taken any medicine or pills of any kind during that time. Then the researchers quizzed the employees in great detail concerning whether they had experienced various symptoms during that three-day period. The symptoms they inquired about were the twenty-five most common symptoms listed as side effects of drugs. They were things like nausea, headache, itching, loose stools, drowsiness, and the like. On close questioning, eighty-seven percent of them admitted to having experienced at least two of the symptoms. The doctors concluded that had the employees been taking a medicine at the time, the medicine would have been blamed for the "side effects." This is one reason why many doctors are reluctant to tell patients about possible side effects. The patient is more apt to have trouble if he knows what to look for. If he is convinced he will have problems, his bio-consciousness has simply been given a blueprint to follow.

People enter the hospital afraid of what the doctors and nurses are going to do to them. This kind of attitude affects healing and recovery and may well produce the very kind of bad result the patient is trying to guard against. We do create our environments. Distrust and fear have the effect of retarding healing, as I explained in the chapter on psychosomatic disease. I believe that most doctors, even ones who could be categorized as mediocre, are capable of practicing better medicine than the majority of patients will allow.

How should patients behave? First of all don't waste the doctor's time with silly, insignificant problems. Statistics show that people who seek medical attention fall into four groups. The first group, consisting of half of all patients, is called the "worried well." These are the people who awaken every morning, look in their throats, stick out their tongues, and feel themselves from top to bottom looking for a lump. When they experience a twinge or an ache, they make a mad dash to the doctor or the emergency room to be assured that they are not about to die. They are not sick. They fear being sick. They are afraid to die, and they are afraid of life. They can't even put enough symptoms together to organize an illness. When I practiced in Illinois, a lot of college professors fell into this category. They were often intellectual snobs you couldn't tell anything to,

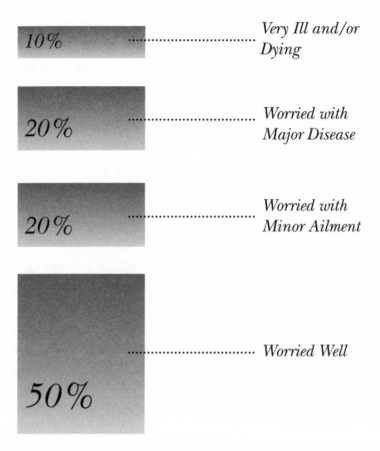

either. These are the individuals whom doctors spend hundreds of millions of dollars on each year, running unnecessary tests. The doctor, fearing a lawsuit for failing to diagnose some illness, is literally forced to perform endless tests to rule out the mere possibility that the "twinge" is the first symptom of some disease.

A second group, making up about twenty percent of patient visits, are worried but also have some minor problem, such as a cold or an infected hangnail, neither of which actually requires the attention of a physician. These people could either treat themselves or wait for whatever is bothering them to go away. Incidentally, most physicians make their living being immediately available to treat patients within a few hours of their first sniffle, or the moment a mosquito bite becomes inflamed.

It is clearly evident that at least seventy percent of all doctor visits are unnecessary. If we are concerned about the cost of medical care in the United States, this might be a good place to start saving.

The third group consists of another twenty percent of the visits. These patients have an illness or a condition for which medical attention is recommended. These are the people with pneumonia, diabetes, high blood pressure, gallbladder attacks, ulcers, broken legs, pregnancy, well baby checkups, and other valid reasons to seek health care. These patients will recover, but the doctor can be of assistance in hastening the recovery, easing discomfort, and perhaps preventing complications.

The remaining people, making up about ten percent, are very sick. Many will never recover from their illnesses, at least not by conventional means, and some of them will die of their conditions. The physician's role, if nothing else, is to help ease these patients' pain and suffering—although most doctors are not very good in this area. They tend to see illness and death as defeat, and thus shy away. They hate to admit that they are not omnipotent. At the metaphysical level of being, illness offers an opportunity to learn, and death is a new beginning.

How should a person conduct himself if something goes wrong? First of all, use common sense. Don't waste the doctor's time with silly problems. *Keep in mind that no one dies or suffers a disability without, on some level, having agreed to have it happen.* I fully realize that this is a bold statement. For it to be made by a physician is nothing less than heresy. Nonetheless, it is true, and for that reason, I have stated it here a number of times. There is no need to go to the doctor with colds, minor cuts, and sprains. If you are wrong in your judgment, you will have adequate time to see the doctor if you are not getting better. Trust your common sense and listen to your inner voice.

Be open and honest with your doctor, telling her all your symptoms and answering her questions with candor. If you do not understand what she is saying, then say so, and ask for a further explanation. If she suggests tests, ask her how she expects the tests to help with the diagnosis or the treatment. When she asks you to return to see her, do so. You can tell if the doctor is actually doing anything or if the visit was wasted and of no importance. Take your medicine as directed. If it seems to make you sick, then call the doctor and check. I had one man with a streptococcal sore throat who quit taking his antibiotic because his fever went higher. In spite of what I told him, he believed that one dose should make him well. So, when his fever rose, he assumed it was a reaction to the medicine and stopped taking it. His action resulted in an abscess that had to be surgically drained.

If you have what appears to be a serious medical problem, do not see the doctor just before noon or at the end of the day, if you can avoid it. There is no question that the quality of medicine practiced at those times of day is inferior to that practiced in the middle of the morning or in the early afternoon. For one thing, being human, the doctor is thinking about lunch or going home for the day. Often at these times, the laboratory and X-ray are not operating at their best, either. Technicians are going to lunch or closing down for the night. Tests ordered then are often scheduled for later, and very often the patient fails to return the next day to get them. In every doctor's practice is a group of patients who choose to come at those times. Invariably, if they have complicated illnesses, they are poorly worked up and inadequately followed. You would not knowingly buy a car that was assembled on Monday morning or the day before a holiday, so do not place yourself in a similar situation with your health care.

The most important thing of all is to assume an attitude of trust and a belief that you are going to recover. You have to go through life trusting someone, and other than your spouse and your kids, I know of no one else better to trust than your doctor. I'm not talking about blind, thoughtless trust in which you allow yourself to be led about by your nose. Use your common sense and judgment.

HOLISTIC MEDICINE

A Different View

WE NOW KNOW that a holistic approach to medical care must first take into consideration the patient. As we have seen, it is the patient who makes contact with the doctor, bringing a multitude of problems into the arena of interaction with the health-care givers. It is the patient who presents us with the illness, and it is the patient who must do the healing. All the medical profession or any other discipline of healing can do is to assist in the process.

I hope that, at this point, it is patently clear that the patient is responsible for getting sick. This is not to place or shift blame, it is just a different and more accurate model of disease than we have been accustomed to thinking about. If medicine is to extend beyond the arena of technical excellence that it has attained today, our society, the public, patients, doctors, therapists, and government agencies, must assume another belief system. We must quit thinking in terms of the ill patient being a victim. In the medical literature, the news, television, magazines, and our common exchange of ideas, we speak constantly of people falling victim to various diseases. We hear about victims of cancer, victims of heart disease, victims of AIDS, victims of high blood pressure, victims of everything.

Throughout this book, I have alluded to the concept that the body is a construct of the spirit. I have hinted repeatedly that it is the soul that has a body and not the other way around. I have intimated that your thoughts are things, as real as rocks and trees, and have the capacity to affect the working of your body. The truth is that our bodies are constantly being constructed according to our thoughts and beliefs. As I have said, the molecules and cells composing the body have a consciousness of their own. They have awareness, intent or purpose, memory, and the ability to communicate. This bio-consciousness follows an electromagnetic thought-blueprint that is given to the cells by the spirit and the genes. In part, this direction comes through the nervous system. (It is actually a far more complex system of communication than this, but thinking of it coming via the nerves is adequate to understanding the process.)

At the same time, your conscious mind is in constant communication with your bio-consciousness, giving it directions other than those received at the outset. And the pattern of directions is constantly being altered by your belief system. Therefore, to a large extent, we grow old simply because we expect to do so. This concept is reinforced constantly, as we watch others about us turning gray, developing wrinkles, walking more slowly, and assuming the changes we associate with growing old. But this does not have to occur. There have been very good, scientifically controlled experiments in which people in their seventies and eighties changed their body physiology to be twenty years younger within the span of a few days (*see* page 74).

In the area of disease, there are thousands of examples of individuals who have been accurately diagnosed as having a terminal illness of one kind or another curing themselves. The methods they used are highly varied, but two things are common to all the spontaneous cures: a focused intent to become healthy again and a clear belief that it is possible to do so. There would be more of these cures except that for an individual to be successful in such a journey, he or she must literally fly in the face of the medical profession and society at large.

I have a close friend who cured himself of a cancer. After the disease had been diagnosed, he did not tell a single soul that he had a cancer or that he had refused medical care. He said his adventure was between himself and the universe and that any outside intrusion, regardless of its good intent, would have been distracting. In general, support groups made up of others who are living the same journey can be very helpful, but in the end, it is a solitary adventure.

To understand more fully the active part the individual plays in developing a disease, it is helpful to understand the spiritual matrix underlying what we consider to be reality. Jane Roberts, in the book *The Individual and the Nature of Mass Events*, talks about a dual framework within the universe. She speaks of Framework 1 as the interaction of personal, social, and physical events with things of which we are aware and in which we work and live in our daily existences. These are the superficial events and actions which we perceive as "real." At the same time that we focus on the events surrounding us, we are in constant contact spiritually through the subconscious with the deeper reality of Framework 2.

Framework 2 is a vast spiritual matrix of relationships, probabilities, fantasy, myth, and imagination made up, in part, by our thoughts and beliefs. It is within Framework 2 that each of us creates multiple dramas of probable life stories. These probable events are real and continue to exist indefinitely, whether we choose to actualize them or not. We select from the myriad possibilities within this framework one that we will actualize. Once actualized, a Framework 2 possibility becomes Framework 1—a part of our daily reality. Because of the intensity of our focus in the superficial Framework 1, we are oblivious to the other probabilities, but they exist and are available to us, even though we did not choose to actualize them into Framework 1.

Many times, we find ourselves locked into hidden assumptions that we chose in childhood or during our teens. As we proceed through life, we continue to react to these hidden assumptions automatically. Frequently, it never occurs to us to reassess our assumptions, much less to change them. Far too often, we are consciously oblivious of them. Thus, as a child, you may have seen your mother die of cancer and childishly assumed the same thing would happen to you. In your world of experience, mothers die at a young age and abandon their families. Such an assumption may become the underlying frame of existence against which all else is of secondary importance. When you reach adulthood, your body dutifully complies with your primary hidden assumption, and you develop a cancer of your own. If you are unaware of this spiritual matrix in which you plan your life, you will perceive yourself as a victim of cancer, never knowing that the malignancy was a result of your childhood belief.

In many ways, life can be thought of as a lighted pathway, one among thousands that lie hidden in the darkness of Framework 2. Out of fear of the unknown, or through ignorance of the existence of those other potential paths, we often plod thoughtlessly and stubbornly along the lighted one, regardless of where it may lead. It takes courage to step off into the darkness and light up an unknown way. The challenge of holistic medicine is to help people recognize that it is possible to take other routes.

In the context of illness, if you choose a line of probability for your life that sees it coming to an end at the age of forty, then subconsciously you will look for a way to end this life and start a new one. You may look to an automobile accident, or if you have a family history of heart disease you have already been given a blueprint for escape. Long before you reach that age, your bio-consciousness will begin to produce the changes in your arteries that will bring about a heart attack at forty. Along the way, if you choose other probabilities from Framework 2 that are in conflict with your departure at age forty, you are free to choose another probability and extend your life. Either the changes in your arteries that were designed by you to bring your life to a close will reverse themselves, or you may be one of those people the doctors talk about, saying, "I don't know what has kept the guy alive all these years. I thought he would have a heart attack twenty years ago."

A person of my acquaintance has been working with a woman who has had a very unfulfilling life with her husband. She has been frustrated in pursuing her own career because she felt tied to him. To become fully involved in her own endeavor would have required her to move to another city. She had come to the point where she needed to make a decision. She could procrastinate no longer, but the decision was not easy. For one thing, if she moved away, she would be perceived as abandoning her husband. There were other considerations as well.

She was relieved of making her choice by a year-long trip to Europe with her husband. She dreaded her return, for she was aware that upon coming home she would finally be forced to decide what she was to do. Shortly before returning to the States, she developed a cough. Upon seeking medical attention, she found she had a cancer of the lung. My friend resumed counseling with the woman. When the subject of her cancer was discussed, the lady said, "You know, when I went to Europe I got off the hook. Now my cancer has done the same thing for me. It's sort of a relief knowing I will not have to make the choice between staying with my husband or going for the career."

At the metaphysical level of existence, cancer represents new growth. It offers an opportunity to explore different lines of probability for the developing soul. In our society, it is very difficult at times to jump from one probable future to another. Very often, the only practical way is to start anew. In the case of the lady with the lung cancer, I am certain that her bio-consciousness created the malignancy for that reason. She was in a deadlock. If she was not going to enjoy her own career, there was little reason to prolong the incarnation. Her cancer was a great gift. On the other hand, she still has a choice. She does not have to die of her cancer. She can choose her career and life. The cancer may well regress and disappear if she comes to grips with its meaning and purpose.

Holistic medicine, if it is to be true to its name, must start with these concepts concerning illness. The medical team must be fully aware of both frameworks. We must abandon the assumption that it is medicine and surgery that cure, for we know that neither does. At the most, they may buy the individual time in which to adopt a new framework. New models of disease must be constructed which allow for different outcomes. The physician must no longer be seen as the central figure in the healing team. He or she is but one of the players and not necessarily even a vital one. The individual in charge who is to work the closest with the patient will be anyone who understands the spiritual-physical aspect of the illness. This person might be a psychic, a psychologist, an acupuncturist, or, perhaps, the doctor.

In the process of healing, the nutritionist will assist by making certain the nutritional state of the body is optimal for healing to take place. The physician needs to stand by in case the individual needs assistance to gain time. For example, if an infection is about to kill a cancer patient, antibiotics can cure the infection and give more time for spiritual reassessment and re-footing to occur. Other technically oriented approaches to health care may from time to time be needed as an adjunct to the healing process. But they should never be thought of as definitive or conclusive.

The main center of activity, for healing to be successful, must revolve around helping the patients form, and then accept, a new belief system and take responsibility for their condition and their eventual outcome. While this new footing is being established, belief in the certainty of the method is of great importance. Therefore, if a particular individual is firmly convinced that surgery or vitamins will secure survival, then those are the methods that must be used. At the same time, the patient must be brought to the point of enlightenment where he or she can see the illness within the perspective of the overall metaphysical view.

This is a picture of holistic medicine at its best. It is not a scenario in which weird doctors do strange things with blinking gadgets and the like. It is a new base of assumption that is as old as the universe. It is not New Age, it is age old. It embraces the spirituality of humankind, empowers us with new vigor, and opens to us new vistas of opportunity.

DEATH AND DYING

ANY BOOK WRITTEN by a doctor should include a few words on death and dying, but many do not. Most physicians even have trouble saying the words out loud, because the very concept conjures up visions of failure. In medical schools, nobody talks very much about patients dying. The situation is generally ignored, as if by our keeping silent death will not occur. At the same time, the message is that doctors are in a constant battle against death, and if the patient dies, the doctor may not have done all that he could. I know that for most of my early years of practice, I felt guilty when one of my patients died. There must have been some test I could have ordered that would have provided me with the information that would have saved the person. Surely some drug or therapeutic measure existed that would have saved my patient if only I had thought of it. I felt responsible for their deaths. Doctors do not like to talk about death.

The truth is that saving lives is not the function of the medical profession, in spite of the fact that doctors believe it to be. Doctors' real purpose is to help patients in their recovery. If death is near, the purpose of the doctor is to recognize the truth of the situation and make death as comfortable as possible. That is a totally different role than most doctors assume. Doctors can prolong the process of dying at times for hours or months, but they cannot prevent death. Physicians sometimes describe their lives as fighting a rear-guard action against death. To this end, they often go to ridiculous extremes. I have seen doctors still writing orders on the chart when the nurse comes to tell them that the patient is dead. The same sort of insanity became even worse when cardiac resuscitation came into general use. Now, dying patients are physically assaulted under the guise of trying to save their lives. No hospital emergency room receives a patient as dead on arrival any longer. Patients are not *allowed* to be DOA. Someone, it seems, has to jump on every patient's chest, shock him, inject all manner of expensive drugs, and place him on a respirator before pronouncing him dead. Partly, this is done out of a misguided attempt to "save" the patient, partly out of a desire to charge a big fee for the heroic effort, and partly in an attempt to avoid a lawsuit.

There is absolutely nothing wrong with dying. People do it every day, and eventually we all will make that glorious adventure. It is true that no one dies before his time, from any cause and regardless of age. It took me almost sixty years to learn that, but learn it I did. Doing cardiac resuscitation in the hospital became so repugnant to me that I walked to the emergency room or the floor where the code was in progress and let the aggressive, uninformed, but wellmeaning medical mechanics dash ahead and take over. Everyone has seen or known of some soul dying of cancer whose life has been filled with pain and misery and who has been put through one or more codes when death finally came. Regardless of the motives involved, such measures are always inappropriate.

As you think back through this book, you'll remember that I have been urging people to take conscious responsibility for their lives. You have been told that the body is a construction of your mind. You have been told that you create your environment and are responsible for the development of disease. You have been told that you shape your own health. Why not, then, accept the final chapter that you orchestrate your own death? Death is not an end. Death is a beginning, just as you might think of birth as your death from the spiritual life from which your soul came before incarnation. When you think about it, birth and death are the same. They are the process in which we change arenas of learning and form.

The mind is a function of the spirit. It exists and thinks whether you are in spirit form or body form. During incarnation, it fuses with the brain and nervous system as a physical vehicle by which it can function. Fused with the brain, it has difficulty remembering its spiritual existence, and as we look back on our childhood and infancy, we have trouble remembering our thought processes as infants. At the time of death, we apparently do not even lose consciousness. Under hypnosis or the recollection of near death experiences, people report times of confusion when they are not aware of death. One young man who recalled being killed in the South Pacific during World War II could not understand why people were not listening to him. It took a while to realize that he had died. Others are immediately aware and proceed to enter the other plane without hesitation. In their book *Life between Life,* Joel Whitten and Joe Fisher have an excellent discussion of the death experience and the activities of souls between incarnations.

From the medical point of view, several things are going to have to change before we will be able to treat the dying with love and grace. First, our culture must assume a different attitude toward life and the universe. We must accept that we are part of an infinite living structure and that we are eternal. Christianity, which colors our thinking in every aspect of this culture, gives lip service to this concept but then denies the validity of what it preaches. We are but sojourners upon the earth, here for only a moment to fulfill a specific purpose. Everyone is fully justified and does not have to be "saved" for any reason. There is nothing to be saved from.

We must grasp the fact that nobody dies or becomes ill who did not plan the event or at least agree to the plan. Then, the medical profession may be able to adopt a new stance. There is plenty for doctors to do without running about all puffed up with their sense of self-importance trying to save lives. This will entail their acceptance of their new role as facilitators of recovery from disease rather than as Physicians who are responsible for the entire process. Last, and equally vital to our new view, the lawyers must get off the back of the medical profession. Even if a doctor has not yet been sued, she hears about suits, and the fear and anxiety are constantly on her mind. Too many lawyers sit in their offices asserting that one person or another should not have died, that the doctor must have done something wrong. And if mistakes were made, they think, then there is nothing wrong with making a profit in the deal.

Everyone is caught up in the false concept that we are victims of disease and accident and the doctor is there for the divine purpose of bringing a cure. Nurses, doctors, lawyers, Aunt Tillie and Uncle Fudd, the next-door neighbor, the bartender, the barber and hairdresser all know this. It is a nice myth, and everyone has accepted it. The problem is that it is not true. Health, illness, accident, recovery, and death are all under the control of each one of us—not the family doctor or the specialist, regardless of his skill or lack of skill. If you become ill, you must accept the responsibility of having the illness for whatever reason. If you get well, that will be at your direction, as well. True, if you have a stupid doctor, he or she might make the recovery a bit more difficult, but recover you will if that is in your plan. Should you choose to die, there is not a single thing your doctor can do about it.

Shocking as these statements may appear, they are a logical outgrowth of the concepts I have introduced throughout this book. Part of our denial of death stems from our almost studied refusal to look inward at the workings and desires of our spirit. We are so focused on the external that we have become blind to anything else. We are consumed with desire to gain power over others, to control the earth, and to possess all we can. We no longer value one another for our honor or integrity, our wisdom and our ability to advise. We are valued, instead, for the things that we own and for our power and influence. We have come to worship—and identify with—almost exclusively our "toys" and possessions. Little wonder that the thought of dying and leaving it all is frightening. Since humankind has all but lost contact with spiritual reality, we are each driven to remain in this plane as long as possible and to cling to every moment of physical life, even when it is filled with agony. The relatives and the doctor know no different, for they, too, are intently focused in this plane while denying any other.

I often think of the death of Socrates as a beautiful thing. True, he had been forced to commit suicide having been falsely accused and found guilty of corrupting youth and preaching a doctrine that made those in power uncomfortable. Nonetheless, the death was handled very well. He was surrounded by his friends and, as the poison took effect, used the event as a vehicle to teach even more lessons concerning life.

As a physician, I have seen death approached in many ways. I have seen families surround the individual with love and support, filling the parting with understanding and regret, much as if they were seeing their loved one off on a long trip. Other families scream, complain, fight, and look for someone to blame. If they cannot focus their frustration against the daughter or son who has been caring for the individual, they direct their anger toward the hospital, the nurses, or the doctor. They make the death an abomination of misdirected intent. They would not think of sending their loved one to the operating room for surgery sobbing and moaning and all the while placing blame. Yet those same people would send their parents into another dimension surrounded by emotional chaos.

Our culture is a long way from handling and approaching death in a mature manner. We are going to have to get in touch with our spiritual being and understand our position in the universe before much will change on a broad scale. Families who have some feeling and knowledge of the infinite must start instructing the medical profession. I have seen relatives look with horror at the tubes, respirators, and other equipment attached to their loved ones. They grimace as the laboratory technician draws still more blood, running the tests the doctor ordered. At the same time, not one has spoken up and said "stop." They look to the doctor to indicate when to accept the inevitability of death, and at times the doctor is hoping for a signal from the relatives that the time is now.

Everyone should talk about terminal illness and how we would like to be treated. A living will with an enduring power of attorney should be made by everyone. It can be written without the help of an attorney and signed with witnesses. Then, the doctor will be legally bound to follow your wishes, even if you become unconscious and unable to state them. Personally, when I die, I do not want someone even thumping on my chest, much less doing a code. If I become ill, and I suppose that one day that might happen, unless I need surgery I have no intention of going to the hospital. I am well aware that I will not die until I am ready. I have made my wishes known to my family. Not long ago, my daughter, who lives some 2,000 miles away, asked what I wanted her to do should I become seriously ill or ready to die. I responded that I expected nothing from her. If she wanted to come and visit, that would be nice, but I do not want her to do so if it is inconvenient. We are both aware of our universal connections and realize that her appearance is unnecessary to indicate her love for me.

The two topics of concern that are least talked about in our culture are sex and dying. We do not handle either well. We cannot prevent death by ignoring it, so we—as a culture—might as well become involved. When children ask about death, they should be told that those who have gone have finished their tasks and learned what they had come here to learn. The children should be told that the dead have gone to prepare for another sojourn on Earth. I believe that they will be back. If your children have been well instructed, telling them that Grandpa went to be with God will seem silly, for they will know that Grandpa has always been with God and did not have to do anything to join the divine. They will one day understand that death and dying are yet another window to enlightenment.

SIXTEEN

FINAL THOUGHTS AND LESSONS

NOT LONG AGO, I met a very uptight young woman at an art show where I was displaying my sculptures. She told me that she, too, was a physician, a specialist in arthritic diseases. We got to talking, and I decided to see how rigidly she was locked into the belief system of conventional medicine. After she had listened to me recount some of the things with which I had been involved, she said, "You never had any direction or consistency in your practice at all. You adhered to nothing!" I looked at her and replied that I had been totally consistent: "Throughout my entire life," I said, "I have been on a quest to acquire wisdom." Her mouth sagged open, and she walked away without even answering.

The entire purpose of individuated human consciousness is to attain wisdom. To the degree that this is done, it allows the individual the opportunity of joining in the creative process of the universe. It is upon the mandate to communicate what I have learned that I base the authority for the statements I have made in this book.

According to my psychic friends and my spiritual guide, I still have another fifty-some years to go. I am looking forward to this, for I want to be around to see what is going to happen to this culture. But personally, I'm scared. We here in the United States don't have much time left. We need desperately to reassess our values and goals. America is like a blind, rich kid dressed in fine clothes and living in a mansion. He can't see where he is going, but he appears to have it all and so the world rushes to follow him. In our rush to acquire things, we have lost our Ground of Being. If we as a nation are to lead the world, we must begin to think for ourselves and assume responsibility for our destiny. To do this, we need to get in touch with the true spiritual entity that is our reality. This does not mean turning to some fundamentalist church or cult, or even going to any church at all. When you think about it, all religions are cults. It doesn't matter whether it is the Roman Catholic Church or the Baptists or the Presbyterians or a Jim Jones or a Branch Davidian wacko from Waco. They all tell you what to believe, how to live, how to think, how to spend your money, and they all are very free when it comes to judging others. We as a nation and a people need to get into touch with our own souls and not feel compelled to relate to any specific dogma or religious belief system.

A vast number of people today do not want to think for themselves. Perhaps it is only that they are afraid to try. In any case, they look to someone to tell them what to believe—just as they look to doctors for the management of their own health. The more dogmatic the experts or the spiritual leaders, the more people there are who flock to hear what they have to say. These pitiful people are not unlike many individuals who remain in the armed services. In exchange for some freedom, the armed services offer security in the form of someone telling you where to go, when to eat, and when to go to bed. Those who join cults are willing to forfeit some of their personal freedom for the security of having a person in authority tell them how to think, what to believe, how to vote, how to conduct their lives, and how to pray.

Other cultures appear to do a far better job than we do when it comes to directing their lives and taking responsibility for their actions. When my wife and I visited China a few years ago, an incident occurred which clearly pointed out a major difference between our cultures. We were scheduled for a boat trip up the Yellow River to see a Buddhist shrine. We rode a bus to the dock where we were to get on a boat, which we found securely anchored in the river, some twenty feet from the dock. The Chinese had solved the problem of boarding very nicely. Two planks, measuring two by ten inches and about ten feet long, had been placed from the dock to several pilings in the river. From there, two more planks spanned the remaining ten feet or so. There was no handrail. The boards weren't even two by twelves. With a gracious bow, we were told to board the vessel. As an added bit of courtesy, a Chinese gentleman smiled and in quite good English said, "Watch your step, prease." All of us walked the planks, which turned out to be quite flimsy. We bounced and swayed and laughed and all of us got aboard. Nobody fell into the river, much to the disappointment of the crowd of grinning Chinese watching the event. I could not help thinking that if this had been the States, none of us would have been allowed to board, even if we had been willing to try. The company operating the cruise would not have taken the risk of one of us falling into the river. Lawsuits would abound.

In China, we all relied on common sense to rule the situation. It was obvious there was a risk involved. We might lose our balance and fall in the water. The planks did not look very sturdy even before we stepped on them. The Chinese would have fished us out if any of us had fallen in the river and offered a sincere apology. They would also have shrugged, saying that falling in the river was a risk we had accepted when we tried to cross the planks. They did not force us to get aboard. The option had been ours.

The fact that we have become a nation of angry crybabies and blame-placers troubles anyone who has read history. No culture, society, or nation can survive if it is unwilling to accept responsibility for its actions and destiny. We dare not continue to look for someone else to blame when things don't go as expected. I have a T-shirt with a slogan: "It isn't whether you win or lose, it's how you place the blame." That pretty well says it all. We have to change now!

Even though it may have sounded as if it were, this is not primarily a book on social change. It is a book on health. Much of what I have written is within the reach of every patient. I have pleaded with you to change your outlook on life. You can change your attitude about health and what to expect from the medical profession right this minute. For those of you who want a "word pill," here are a few more directions grouped together in one place, a few more things to do that will change your life and health.

First, do not go to any doctor who will not talk to you. Of course, doctors are busy and haven't the time to discuss at length every little problem, but if you are truly concerned and have some questions, you should get some straight answers. If the doctor is honest enough to tell you when he or she is uncertain about a diagnosis, cooperate so that the doctor has a reasonable chance to do what is necessary to make the diagnosis. If it is necessary to call a consultant, the doctor is in a better position to determine who can be of the most help. It is important that doctors are able to work together in harmony. If you choose a consultant with whom your doctor is unable to work, then you have placed yourself at a disadvantage.

You need to treat your body so that the powers of healing and regeneration have an environment with the proper raw materials to effect those processes. Avoid the use of tobacco, alcohol, and addicting street-type drugs. Eat as balanced a diet as possible, most of the time. Then, for heaven's, if not your own, sake, take a good comprehensive vitamin-mineral supplement.

There is no need to run to the doctor for prescriptions for common remedies. Dozens of excellent medicines are available over the counter in every drugstore in the country. Most of them were prescription drugs a few years ago and work as well now as they did then. Let your pharmacist assist you if you're not sure. Keep in mind that new medicines are not necessarily better.

As I have stated before, not every cut, scratch, or minor sprain requires medical attention. I have had patients run to my office to have a cut no more than a half-inch long fixed. When I applied a Band-Aid, they were disappointed I had not sewed them up. For a Band-Aid, they paid for an office visit! You need to trust your common sense. Many of you haven't used it for such a long time that it's probably rusted, but shine it up and start practicing. Your subconscious mind knows when to seek professional help.

If you have one of the chronic diseases I listed in the chapter on maladaptive food reactions, try testing yourself with the various foods you eat on a regular basis. If you become weak holding some food, eliminate it from your diet. If you get better, then eat it again and see if the disease flares up. If it does, then quit eating that food. Try it. What do you have to lose?

You should buy the book *Touch for Health* by John F. Thie. Dr. Thie is a chiropractor, and his book can be very valuable in balancing your acupuncture meridians. It gives some other very basic, simple things to do that can also help a lot. Incidentally, if you pull your back muscle lifting something or wake up with a stiff neck, a visit to a chiropractor makes more sense than going to a medical doctor. The chiropractor will help you. The medical doctor will just give you pills until your body gets well on its own.

Again—I repeat and repeat—people must start thinking for themselves! We are constantly bombarded by advertising and public service announcements designed to frighten us into turning to some "expert" in order to know what to think and do. A recent television commercial for a soap containing a chemical designed to kill bacteria is a good example. The product itself is misleading, once you recognize that soap kills bacteria all by itself and does not require the addition of some special chemical. The commercial's plea comes from a frantic mother proclaiming she must protect her family from the germs that are everywhere! We must have some magic soap, if the ad is believed, otherwise we will drop like flies from some dread disease spread by germs. That's why you have an immune system, and, besides, most bacteria do not cause illness. These advertisements prey upon the fears of an ignorant public that has accepted the premise that they are powerless to help themselves. What is worse is that while they implant these fears to sell their products, advertisers render people more susceptible to infection. Undirected, nonspecific anxiety does nothing, except make the individual more prone to the very thing it fears. For that matter, making the common signs of cancer known to people may very well increase the incidence of those very cancers.

Many years ago, I used to take my turn working in the emergency room of the local hospital. I was appalled by the number of people who failed to trust their own instincts and common sense. It was fairly common to see someone who had been in a car accident. Although many did not have a single bruise, bump, pain, scrape, or scratch anywhere on their bodies, they insisted upon being X-rayed to see if they had been hurt. When people constantly run to the doctor with minor complaints and symptoms, they are headed for trouble. If they persist long enough, some doctor will help them find an illness. That's what doctors do. They keep searching until they find something wrong. They are trained to diagnose disease, not wellness. Most doctors don't even know what wellness is. Go to an internist week after week, and she will order endless tests and prescribe tons of pills. Take a complaint to a surgeon and go back often enough with it and sooner or later you will end up with an operation. That's what surgeons are trained to do. They cut people open and take things out.

In the United States, we have come to think that life must be totally comfortable, pain and disease free, and affluent. And of course we must remain forever thin, never get wrinkles, and never die. There is no rule that says people cannot work feeling sick or with their backs hurting. Expectations and beliefs that people must be perfectly healthy and comfortable are totally unrealistic, yet the doctors, because of the expectations of the patients, must work within this frame of belief at all times. This belief system also creates more business for the doctors, so they are not about to tell you differently.

Seeing older patients complaining of osteoarthritic pain in their knees is a common occurrence in the United States. One day, I asked a friend how he handled these cases? He was an excellent orthopedic surgeon who was born and raised in Europe. He went to medical school and practiced in his native country for several years. Since he was a specialist, I thought he might have some approach to therapy that was better than what I had to offer.

He said he had no special approach to the problem. Every day he saw six or seven older people in his office complaining bitterly of the arthritic pain in their knees. He went on to add that in all his years practicing in Europe he could not remember a single patient with such a complaint. I was confused and inquired if they did not get osteoarthritis. He assured me the folks in his native country got arthritis the same as they did here in the United States. He concluded by saying that it did not occur to the people there to complain about it. Older people with pain due to osteoarthritis accepted the pain and discomfort as part of growing old, part of life and aging.

In Japanese plays, the comedy character is often an old man who complains about his misfortunes. He will cry, saying his house burned down, and the audience roars with laughter. He will moan and groan that he lost his fortune, and again the audience laughs. In Japan, it is assumed that age is accompanied by maturity and wisdom. For an old man to be complaining about the misfortunes of life is, to them, totally absurd and truly funny. Life is life. It is to be accepted and dealt with in the most appropriate way possible.

As a culture, we have deluded ourselves into expecting that everything should be perfect, and if it is not, we look about for someone or something to blame. Every once in a while you hear on the news that some toy has been taken off the market because it is unsafe. Certainly toys should be reasonably safe, the paint should be non-toxic and all that. Not long ago, I heard a news commentator say that a toy was being recalled because there were some rough edges that might possibly cause a child to be cut. I was reminded of all the toys I had with sharp edges. I got cut, scratched, and pinched from time to time. I didn't lose any fingers, and I don't know of a single kid who ever did. Those minor injuries taught me a lot. I learned what sharp edges can do, not from being warned, but from firsthand experience. I learned to be careful. I learned that a minor cut sometimes did not even need to be bandaged, much less require my going to the doctor with it. I learned to observe things, looking for a place where I might be pinched or scratched. I'd show them to my father and he'd file them smooth. Later, I fixed them myself. I started to learn to use tools. At some point in life, one has to learn how to handle sharp things without getting cut. What better time to do it than when we are kids? Native American children, I'm told, were never prevented from crawling into the fire in the center of the teepee and getting a finger or two burned. The children were not neglected. On the contrary, they were closely watched. The parents reasoned, however, that they would have a better appreciation of "hot" if they experienced it. Once burned, the kids were very careful around the fire.

If your child cuts his finger off on his toy "Whatsit" or falls from the swing set breaking his neck, it was planned somewhere. Perhaps it was her karma at work for her own instruction or maybe it happened for your benefit, so why sue someone? I did hypnosis on a man who believed that, as a boy, he had once been killed by a freight wagon. His death had been for the instruction of his mother and father, he said. They needed to learn how to deal with the loss of a child. Whatever the case, such deaths are certainly not arranged by the gods in order for the parents to sue the freight companies and make bundles on the loss of their children.

One of the underlying themes of this book is to relax and enjoy life. Revel in the trials and tribulations. Remember, good times are defined by tough times, just as up defines down, and light, dark.

If, for example, there were no such thing as down, there could be no concept of up. "Up" implies there must be some place that "up" is from. This is an ancient concept of Tao, the law of opposites. Opposites do not oppose one another; they define each other.

Parenting has changed a lot through the years. I was ill quite a bit when I was a boy, with infected ears, sinus infections, and strep throats. As I look back, some of my fondest memories were when I was ill. I was always close to my parents, and we expressed our love openly, saying "I love you," and patting, and hugging, and kissing. But the sick times were special. Mom would paint my throat with cotton swabs soaked in Mercurochrome, and both my parents would give me alcohol rubs to bring my temperatures down. Dad was especially good at holding my head in his hands to help the pain of my headaches. These were special times of love and caring. Nowadays, too many kids miss out on all these expressions of true parental concern.

Throughout this book, I have criticized the medical profession rather harshly. It is only fair that I offer some solution or plan for the betterment of the healing professions. The problem with attempting to offer a solution for improving health care in this country is that solving it is like untying the Gordian knot of Phrygia, and I fear the solution may not be unlike that used by Alexander the Great.

Health care costs are eating us alive. It wouldn't be so bad if they truly were "health care costs," but they are, instead, *crisis care costs.* Efforts to control the runaway expenses will fail because, if that is all we attempt to do, we will start at the wrong end of the problem. Paying for crisis care for everyone in the country is not the answer and will bankrupt the nation. If health care were directed at preventive care and based upon a different view of the nature of humankind, it would be far more effective.

There are other fundamental issues that must be faced, as well:

- *Doctors are directly responsible, in one way or another, for the vast majority of the money spent on health care. Therefore, in some fashion, the doctor's income must be affected if he or she persists in ordering useless tests, hospitalizing folks when they do not require it, and performing unnecessary and inappropriate procedures.*

- *The patients and their families must face the fact that it is all right to die. Dying is a normal thing to do.*
- *The public has to be educated to change their belief that they must see a physician every time they get an ache or a twinge.*
- *Let us help the "worried well" handle their problems rather than "being taken care of" and insisting the doctor fuss over them, running countless tests.*

In order to redirect crisis care to health care in an effective fashion, I propose that the president appoint a national task force to study the delivery of health care in the United States. The task force should comprise two individuals from each of the following disciplines: allopathy, dentistry, chiropractic, homeopathy, psychology, acupuncture, nutrition, and nursing, as well as two nonprofessionals and, last of all, two psychics. The individuals chosen to represent their fields should probably not be professors holding staff positions in teaching institutions, since they are more likely to be steeped in convention and too rigid to be dispassionate evaluators of their respective fields. The members of the commission should be recognized as masters in their respective fields but must be known to be free of convention.

They should be given a specific time frame in which to work. In the first two years, they should identify and pool knowledge and treatments that are truly valid and effective from each of the disciplines. They should then determine the common truths binding these seemingly diverse pieces of knowledge and various therapeutic approaches into an integrated whole.

Another year would be utilized to develop a statement or position paper upon the nature of humankind and its relation to the universe and on how that relationship affects health and disease. In other words, the commission should begin by outlining another belief system that incorporates a different view of humanity, as well as different concepts of the causes and treatment of non-health. The new belief system contained in the position paper should be taught in all classes of every health-care related school in the country, and the schools should be required to accomplish this paradigm change within a two-year period, thus completing the entire process. From the forming of the commission to implementation of the new concepts should require no more than a span of five years.

This is not so far-fetched a proposal. In about 1910, the Flexner report resulted in just such a thing. Curricula of medical schools were standardized and schools were graded. If the schools were to gain federal support and the students were to have equal status in licensure, they had to conform to the findings of the Flexner study and alter their academic teaching.

But to accomplish this, the government must quit turning to the medical profession for all the answers. It is interesting that we have a Surgeon General to advise the president in health matters. Why not a Psychologist General or a Chiropractor General or a Dentist General or even a Psychic General? The AMA represents a minority of health-care practitioners, and when one adds up all the individuals other than allopathic physicians who administer health care, it is obvious that the AMA represents a small minority, indeed.

If we are not to be required to wait a century or more for a truly eclectic health-care system to evolve, some organization with the power of the federal government must become involved and make a beginning. Such a commission as I have proposed could truly open a new era. Personally, I believe the public is ready. It may have been so for quite a long time.

But the AMA is not ready. It never will be. Its members are so dedicated to their own vested interests that anything they say must be suspect. In spite of this, I believe many health-care practitioners are ready to strike out in an attempt to discard the cobwebs and moss of convention but are prevented from doing so by peer pressure and fear of litigation. Change will constitute a true revolution, and, knowing the medical profession as I do, a revolution may be the only way to accomplish the task.

Then, in some fashion short of shooting them all, we must get the lawyers off the backs of the doctors. Let us return malpractice litigation to actual cases of malpractice where the doctor has been shown to be grossly negligent rather than the legal rip-off it has become in the last generation. Lawyers do not have to prove anything any longer; they simply have to *allege* that the doctor did something wrong, file a suit, and the insurance companies will pay off a few thousand just to get the case settled.

If you have been paying attention, it is obvious that I believe the doctor plays only one part in the process of recovery from illness. Throughout this book, I have said that the body constantly receives instructions from the subconscious mind and that recovery depends upon the attitude of the patient. It is inaccurate and totally unfair to place the entire burden of recovery at the feet of the doctor. As I have said, patients often do not comply with the directions of the doctor, yet I have never heard of a patient getting on the witness stand in a malpractice suit and admitting that she did not follow directions. The legal profession has become wealthy by instilling in everyone the concept that we are victims of whatever may befall us. It is always more comfortable to blame someone else for your misfortune, and, far too often, it becomes profitable to do so.

I have seen excellent doctors ruined by a frivolous malpractice suit in which the jurors admitted later that, though they did not think the doctor had been negligent, they had ruled out of sympathy for the patient. They reasoned that the doctor's insurance would pay the settlement and that he would not be hurt. Little did they know the effect upon his spirit. One highly skilled and conscientious orthopedic surgeon I knew personally almost quit practice after being found "guilty" when he had slaved and agonized for weeks attempting to save his patient's leg. The patient had been riding a motorcycle at a high speed and dead drunk when he hit a tree, fracturing his leg in no less than eight places. Experts testified that the surgeon had done everything possible. But the jury awarded the patient one million dollars, not because they felt the doctor had done something wrong, but because they felt sorry for the poor man. Naturally, the lawyer pocketed half of the settlement. Not a bad bit of change for nearly ruining a doctor's confidence and career.

In truth, the most any patient can expect from a doctor is some help from time to time. The recovery is in the hands of the patient, and, unless the doctor prescribes a fatal dose of some drug or performs some other obviously stupid and harmful act, his part in the eventual "bad result" is amazingly small. This is not something the legal profession wants to hear, but it is correct.

The main thing you must accomplish if you wish to turn your life around, whether it is your health or your relationship with the universe, is to adopt a different attitude. If things do not seem to be changing, then sit down with yourself and do some soul searching. Perhaps for some reason you do not wish life to be different. Perhaps you would rather have someone to blame than accept the fact that the circumstances you are complaining about are of your own making. Start examining your basic assumptions about life and health. It may well be that you are acting on some beliefs that are not consistent with what you would choose at this point in time. If so, then set about altering them by choosing another line of probability from Framework 2.

Look about you. The world is populated with humans, animals, and plants that are your companions in life. Treat every single one of them as if your very life depended upon a loving and cooperative sharing of the universe—because it does. The universe is a living creature, and you are just a very small part of the system. To the degree that we destroy other species, we lessen the richness of the totality of the universe and the quality of our spiritual existence.

Last of all, there are probably more good, honest doctors of all kinds out there who are interested in alternative health care methods than either of us knows about. Feel your doctor out. If he gets hostile or defensive, then maybe he isn't the doctor for you. If your doctor is not aware of some of the things I have addressed in this book, then ask him why he does not know about them. Indicate that you are interested in having him try some alternate approach, especially if you are not doing awfully well with the standard methods. There is no reason that he cannot read something other than the accepted medical journals. There isn't a single good reason why he cannot question some of the things he has been taught that are obviously of little value. On the contrary, it is every doctor's duty to do so.

As you read—and, I hope, re-read—this book, there may appear to be a number of contradictions. In one place, I tell you that illness is a result of an immature attitude toward life; in another, bad nutrition; and elsewhere, some food reaction or your own thinking. Contrary to appearance, these are not opposing concepts. All the factors mentioned in the book may be at work at different times—or all at once. One of the major difficulties in writing this book was to separate the concepts into chapters. This should be evident from the way my chapters overlap. New perspectives need to be presented several times and in many different ways.

I have offered a number of different concepts and beliefs which I personally consider to be irrefutable. Through my forty-four years as a practicing physician and sixty-nine years of this life experience, they have stood up to testing innumerable times. I felt it important to share them with you.

Do I have all the answers? Certainly not! I have learned only a small bit of truth—a nibble at the edge of the big cookie of knowledge. At some point, when I step into another dimension of life and reality, I intend to have all the answers. But I know that will be an impossibility then, too. As a tiny bit of this living entity we call the universe, I know the universe is continually evolving, recreating itself, developing, and maturing. Answers that are valid today are not infinite, for in the future they will be obsolete. But truths do not become untruths, any more than your tricycle ceased to be a valid mode of transportation. It still works. You could ride it to work every day if you chose. You have simply outgrown your tricycle. It was replaced by your bicycle and now your car. An automobile is no more valid a means of transportation than a tricycle; it is just more evolved. So it is with knowledge.

I am not going to say—like Will Rogers—that I never met a man I didn't like. I've met some people who were a real pain in the neck, some who were mean, dishonest, and disgusting, but I learned from them all. Sometimes, it was a lesson I wasn't real keen on learning. But it was a lesson, nonetheless. Many of the people I have met have been doctors, and I have learned a great deal from them, some good and some bad. I would like to think that the majority of the doctors mean well and have the best intentions to treat their patients with skill and compassion. I don't really know whether those doctors make up the bulk of the medical profession or not. Some of the physicians I have known have been great human beings and truly deserved my admiration and that of their patients. It is always easier, however, to remember the others.

After reading this book, you should come away with a better understanding of your nature. I hope you will begin to sense that you are a part of a living universe, not separate from it, and to sense further that the universe and God are one. As a part of this living Being, you will see your body as more than a flesh-and-blood mechanical device. You will see a dynamic energy field, constantly changing within a greater energy field that is also evolving and at all times reflecting your thoughts. What is more, you should know your true self as a spirit. During this time of your existence, you are fused with an energy field of your own construction, which you call a body. Your spirit uses your brain to think and remember. Furthermore, every cell composing that body has consciousness, thinks, remembers, and conforms to your wishes.

Realize that you are in complete control of your life. You are the creator of your own truth.

Sit down once in a while and talk to a rock or a tree. They are both alive, and if you really listen—not with your ears but with your heart—you may perceive them talking back to you. When that happens, you haven't gone over the edge, you have just gotten in touch with the universe.

Life in this incarnation is momentary. It takes place in the eternal NOW. Enjoy it. Don't borrow trouble.

In *The Tao of Pooh*, Winnie the Pooh was asked about people who constantly run about seeking rewards and meaning through various activities and endeavors—out beyond the rainbow. You know, the grass is always greener . . . . Pooh answered something to the effect that those who look for the great reward out beyond the rainbow burn their toast a lot.

As I ponder my years of practice and the thousands of patients I attended, I am not certain the medicines I prescribed were of much value. What I did was attempt to lead my patients to an understanding of themselves. I tried a lot of different ways, whatever seemed appropriate. I talked a lot and taught a lot. With some I reasoned; with others I begged and pleaded. I told stories and jokes to illustrate the points I was trying to make. Occasionally, I used insults, yelled, pounded the desk, or swore. I used every approach I could think of to get my patients involved and to force them to accept responsibility for themselves, their treatment, and their recovery. Perhaps, in the long run, the most important thing I did was to love them.